Discovering Your Inner Style

8 Steps to
G.U.R.U.

by

Jan Addams MIRM

Image to Interior™
Vancouver, BC, Canada

National Library of Canada Cataloguing in Publication Data
Addams, Jan, 1959–
Discovering your inner style: 8 steps to G.U.R.U.

ISBN 0-9781248-0-4

1. Beauty, Personal. 2. Clothing and dress. 3. Interior decoration.
4. Identity (Psychology) I. Title.

BF637.S4A375 2006   646.7
            C2006-903967-4

Cover Design: Cathrine Levan, KickStart Communications Inc.
Artwork: Cale G. Atkiinson, Getty Images, Broderbund
Layout: Cathrine Levan, KickStart Communications Inc.

Copyright © 2006 Jan Addams

Published by:
Image to Interior Inc.
Vancouver, BC Canada

Printed and Bound in Canada
First printing: September, 2006

10 9 8 7 6 5 4 3 2 1

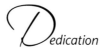

$\mathcal{D}$edication

I dedicate this book with love to my family, my sons Michael and Ryan Addams who have loved me unconditionally and understood my need to search for my own truth.

While becoming my authentic self, some very incredible career and personal paths have occurred. This journeying has led me to the doors of many talented and wonderful people including my amazing husband, Glen Atkinson, who has tirelessly helped bring my dreams to life.

I would also like to thank my extended family and friends for loving me as I was, as I am and giving me the courage to grow into the next version of me.

Thank you all from the bottom of my heart!

Just Jan

Acknowledgements

Anyone having had the opportunity to work on a large project knows that it is never a one person job. A catalyst with vision is absolutely necessary to start, but to bring the dream to life it takes a team of dedicated, like-minded individuals.

The cliches of "Misery loves company", and "Joy shared is doubled", is truly experienced upon the completion of a job well done. I have been blessed with just such a group. These people are highly intelligent, creative, and professional. They have done much more then their "work". They have been leaning posts in times of uncertainty, support when I have been discouraged and just plain tired. These wonderful people include my sister, Judy who mothered me through many life pains, Sheryn and Ward Krywolt, Richard and Virginia Will, Bob and Ellie Laird, Dale and Brenda Johnson, Sandra and Bob Meredith, Sherry Borshiem, Laurel Hillton, Susan Wong, Dawn Andre, Debra Reynolds and Cale Atkinson my amazing artistic buddy who created each chapter's style cartoon.

Thank you to all my "Insider Tips", contributors Kim Pettifer of pHresh Spa, Mary Campeotto of Boccoli Hair and Helen Sergiannidis of Pretty Girl, for their words of wisdom and advice on style and image enhancement.

I would especially like to thank my cheerleader agent, Cathrine Levan of KickStart Communications, for giving my book a fresh new look, and for for her relentless determination to push this project to the finish line when I wanted to quit.

$\mathcal{F}$oreword

"People often say that 'beauty is in the eye of the beholder,' and I say that the most liberating thing about beauty is realizing that you are the beholder. This empowers us to find beauty in places where others have not dared to look, including inside ourselves." -Salma Hayek

I heartily agree! Look into the eyes of a new mother, holding for the first time, her little wrinkled bundle of joy. As their eyes lock, the secret revealed is that each are looking at the most beautiful vision they have ever seen. As women who have experienced motherhood, we feel intense love for the baby we nurtured inside of us for nine months. However, we seldom allow ourselves a fraction of that same unconditional love for our own inner child.

Discovering Your Inner Style started as my own personal journey. With over 30 years of unveiling secrets, I find the information I continue to discover as valid today as it was back then. You see, I, like most women looked in the mirror and saw only my faults. Led by the media's version of beauty, I felt woefully inadequate. I now believe that "beauty is much more than skin deep".

In the process of trying to fix my external façade to meet the beauty standards of the day, I looked at the bigger picture by traveling inward. I discovered an inner character that conflicted with my clothing style due to misconstrued beliefs. I now, however, wear the colours and styles that enhance my face and body shape. I resolved my style conflicts and created a foolproof wardrobe that expresses my style. This is what I want to share with you to help you create your own unique style.

I am a real, passionate, loving and creative person just like you.

My name is Jan........Just Jan

$\mathcal{P}$reface

We have all spent countless time and money on compromises. It is time to educate and then learn to trust our inner voice. "But how?" you ask. There are so many choices, so many conflicting theories. Where does one draw the line?

There is hope. I have discovered some common denominators within those theories that I guarantee will make your consumer life much easier. This and the next two upcoming books in the Triple ID Style Classification © series; Discovering Your Interior and Industry Style can be used as your basic A B C building blocks to build your own personal style.

This book will discuss, analyze and simply solve the following concepts and theories:

1. Inner-Traits – discovering your own strengths and weakness and understanding others to make use of the Platinum rule. "The Platinum Rule" by Dr. Tony Alessandra PhD, CSP, CPAE

2. Colour Analysis – Learn how to effectively use colour to enhance you.

3. Body Shapes – marrying your bone structure with your personal image

4. Interior Design "Style Shapes"– design dominoes will be explained in the next book, due out in 2007. *Discovering Your Interior Style*, will remove the confusion put in place by the use of style terms like Contemporary, Modern, Traditional, Country, Eclectic and Romantic and replace them with easily understandable, useable and recognizable style shapes.

Take the information inside this book test it, experiment with it, and then expand upon it. Don't be intimidated by the cover models you see on the news stands. Or, the decorating shows that mislead you into thinking that by removing all your treasured items, considered clutter, and quickly changing your space into the latest look or trend you will experience ultimate satisfaction.

The information given in this book is by no means a fad diet or a quick fix. This is real, life changing knowledge that will bring out the Guru in you. For that matter, look at the word GURU and spell it aloud. Gee – U – R – U! By the time, you finish the book you will be your own image and interior design GURU and will become the real, authentic you, *Inside* and *Out*!

If you're like me, you've probably explored ways to make yourself look and feel healthier, prettier and more comfortable in your own skin. Maybe you have or, are still searching for that perfect life mate, home or career. Possibly you have felt the need to become better educated and more financially secure. Or, maybe you have come to the point of reinvestigating your deeper, spiritual side.

Well, I have too. In fact for more than thirty years, I have been become a personal and spiritual development information sponge. You see, I started on a personal inward journey, desperately trying to figure out who I was. I asked family. I asked friends. I asked the Church. I received the standard answers, a pat on the head and was told, "Don't worry, have faith." But faith wasn't answering my questions, and I had many.

I started to read books and attend classes on subjects that always interested, but also confused me. I thought that if I could physically see whatever the "bee in my bonnet" was at that time, there would also be someone who knew the answers to my questions, right? Wrong! I was only beginning to find out how wrong that assumption was. As I looked around, I realized I wasn't alone in the wilderness of conflicting ideals and theories.

This led to several years where I questioned and studied everything from ideals to design theory and concepts. Inside this book you will discover as I did, some of the hidden answers to your inner doubts.

Table of Contents

$\mathcal{I}$ntroduction

The information you are about to read is tried, tested and true knowledge that has been revised numerous times for ease of understanding and effortlessness application. I guarantee that with this new awareness, you will accept, respect, love and bring forth the - *Real* - *Live* - *Now* - *And True You* for the entire world to see! The following four fields of study are: personality or innertraits, personal and industry colour use, body shapes and designing your G.U.R.U. style.

Personality Traits: Your Innertraits

Have you ever encountered people that acted either like bulldogs or like milquetoasts? I have run into both. The bulldog types wanted to bite me off at the knees wherein I reacted in one of two ways: either, I rapped them on the nose, or I ran away as if my life depended on it! I learned later, that I reacted as I did depending on the strength or inner power I felt at the time - but that is a whole other topic!

My search began by trying to find out the mysteries of why people act and react the way they do. Wow, the books on that subject! Theories that relate weak areas in the body to causing our personality quirks - "Choleric, Melancholy, Sanguine", and "Phlegmatic" were often used to describe the four basic personality types.

Other books or courses give modern names to the same four personality types. Some of the new terms are Driver, Analytical, Talker, and Watcher; or another course refers to them as Director, Thinker, Socializer, and Relator, or if you have studied Astrology, the elements Fire, Air, Water, and Earth describe pretty much the same traits. There are many books on the subject of personality traits. Of course, little twists and turns make the modern theories seem like new insights.

I to, have taken bits and pieces from each train of thought. Planner Doer, Mediator and Communicator relay similar, but more simplified information about our core personality or innertraits.

I was searching for **Truth** – the whole truth and nothing but the truth – until I realized truth is what is right for you at a particular moment in time. I had finally begun to understand that even truth evolves – our truth, that is. My next curiosity dealt with the phenomenon of colour

Personal and Industry Colour Use

As an Interior Designer and amateur artist, colour has always fascinated me. I noticed early on that some friends looked better wearing some colours, but not others. I too, felt comfortable around certain colours and edgy around others. I bet you can guess what was coming in vogue, having *your colours done.*

First came the 4 Seasons colour theory, then the Time of Day colour theory. Mass confusion and I was in the middle of it! I had thought the teachings of Johannes Itten (who used three primary colours as base to mix all the rest), or Albert Munsell (who gave us the five primary colours evenly distributed around a circle, displaying various intensities of each hue) was complicated enough but some of these new theories made their work seem simple!

My life has always been centered around colour. I have helped hundreds of people with their interior and personal colour choices. I am still constantly amazed at the effectiveness of proper colour treatment and placement be it used on a person or in an interior space. Because I saw the total frustration that my clients went through when choosing the right colour for their wardrobe or interior, I designed a simple to use and apply colour ruler system call Colour Harmonics with a patented colour tool by the same name. In Step 2 you will learn how to personally distinguish, use and apply this system.

Body Types

Being an observer of people, and frustrated with my own body, body types – became my next field of study. Let us see, there was a theory on your body type determined by what kind of food you craved. Another stated that the predominant gland in your body controlled your shape. Of course, there was always a new diet or exercise program promising to change you into the ultimate model shape! The trouble was even though these theories contained some truth and were somewhat valid in their claims how did this knowledge help me to feel better about who I was right now? Instead, I found all this new information gave me one more thing to worry about! Was there no one around who knew how to work with our existing body, without trying to change it into something different?

Again, I was looking for answers and some consistency. On my quest, I discovered that each body shape seem to display different and yet consistent tendencies that showed up in their innertrait responses, clothing and furniture style selections. You will discover in Step 3 how to assess and begin to love your own body shape's uniqueness.

Creating Your Own Design Style

By birth or by curse, I am an interior design merchandiser. The sheer complexity of this field has driven me to create the Triple ID Style Classification System© which incorporates how your innertraits, personal colouring, and body shape merge into your interior design. This book deals with the first three aspects and briefly touches on how your inner style merges into your interior design style for a total look.

You will find a great resource for applying your personal style in the upcoming *Discovering Your Interior Style - 8 Steps to Design Diva*. I've also included a list of suggested reading on all related topics on page 174. Remember that my original purpose for studying these topics was to find myself and simplify my life. In doing so, I felt maybe - just maybe - all that I've gone through in search of me can help others find themselves, with a lot less pain and confusion than I went through.

Time to consult the mirror...............

Looking at "The Big Picture"

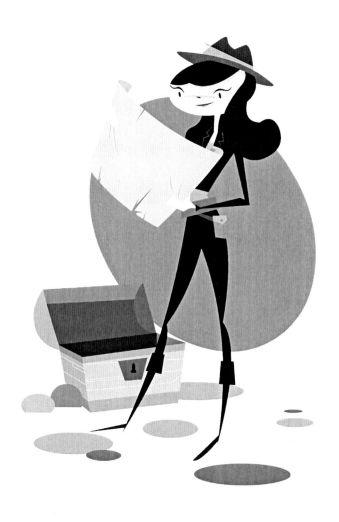

Love and Life
Black and White

Sun and Moon
are Husband and Wife

We wish for strength
We want for might
Why do we live in so much strife?

We climb the hill
We walk the dale

Knowing inside, we cannot fail
Clambering on both day and night
To find our blessed Birth Right!

We search hither
We search far

Ending our search back where we are
Realize our answers don't
come from without
Our answers are inside,
behind the doubt!

Happy Journeying

Looking at the "Big Picture"

Many stories of the universe and world history have relayed discontent with oneself and one's neighbour since the beginning of time. Science, philosophy and religion have tried to shed light on our origins and are still at odds with how we actually got here (though each belief structure holds much passion behind its own version of origin).

So it appears that in the beginning of consciousness an awareness of oneself emerged and with that a natural curiosity of self-comparison to others. Fish wanted to walk on land, monkeys saw the need to become man, gods wanted to enjoy physical pleasures and the bible's Adam needed company and viva la difference! Which leads us to today.

Mirror, Mirror on the wall.......
Do you have a certain model-like image that you aspire to become before you allow yourself to feel great? Close your eyes and picture this image. Now, erase it!

It is my hope that the information I am going to share with you will change in a positive way, the view you have of yourself and your life. I wish for you to become the truly unique human being you are inside and out.

> Do you have a certain model-like image that you aspire to become before you allow yourself to feel really great?

Information abounds on how to improve ourselves. However, most books start from the premise that you are not good enough as you are and therefore you need to change and here is how you can do it. Few people take action on what they read unless they have a burning desire to change. Translation: *The pain of not changing is greater then the pain created from making the necessary change.* - Anthony Robbins

I personally reached the point where everything I held sacred and judged as truth was no longer valid. If you have ever encountered this, you will understand the great void left in your life.

In this age of mass communication, we are knowledge rich, but wisdom poor. Minds full, but bodies inactive. I believe that we all must come to the point of questioning our closely held viewpoints and uncover their roots. If you have let others decide what was good for you in the past, it is time to stop and question their motives, then yours for listening to them.

Confront yourself with the age-old question – Who am I? This question, if taken as far as possible, will allow you the slack you need to say I am human with two arms and legs, five senses (working on the sixth, seventh and eighth), feelings, hopes and dreams. I am not perfect but that's OK! I am who I am. There is only one of me and I'm a good, kind, somewhat misunderstood (by others and myself) *Human Being!"*

This process is not necessarily wonderful. In fact, sometimes you will feel like you are in a dinghy in the middle of the ocean, with no land in sight! However, upon arrival at this stage in our human development we will then be able to take charge of our own lives.

> This book is based on an adapted understanding of the theory of Yin and Yang.

Glamour magazines, decorating books, and how to television shows create the illusion that our clothes, job, vehicle we drive and interior design style defines us. They do, to a certain degree. Unfortunately nobody can agree on what that looks like, and we end up in a never-ending sea of confusion.

So, from the very beginning of this book you will understand why you do things the way you do and learn to love your body, face and hair by wearing clothing, make-up and hairstyles that flatter and enhance your shape. All these components are explored to allow you the personal freedom to be yourself.

Be aware that whether you are refreshing your style, or doing a complete makeover, these physical activities are really the external manifestation of your internal mental, emotional and even spiritual change. I personally have experienced this change and have helped many clients go through their own shifts. This book is based on an adapted understanding of the theory of Yin and Yang. That being the combination of *Finite & Infinite* flowing to *Balance* or *Harmony* creating a new creature *Ying!*

Yin and Yang are dependent opposites that must always be in balance. They appear in print as two entities in a circle but they are actually 3D components of a sphere. These opposites flow in a natural cycle replacing the other. Yin and Yang are explained as a duality that cannot exist without both parts.

> Just as in winter, a seed lays in wait to become life, so it is that Yang waits within Yin for its turn to flow.

Within Yang, there is a small piece of Yin. Within Yin, there is a small piece of Yang. Just as in winter, a seed lays in wait to become life, so it is that Yang waits within Yin for its turn to flow.

There are things in life that are set or *finite* ie: the sun rising, gravity, seasons, etc. Other things continue to evolving or are infinite ie: weather conditions, population growth, etc. And so it is with us. Some parts of our makeup are inherent and others are *creative evolution* as it were.

Our Inner Characteristics

There are common denominators that stay with us throughout our life, and aspects of our personality that change with experience and maturity. By first knowing how you act and react, you then have a basis for understanding and getting along with others.

There Are 4 Basic Personality Traits or Inner-Traits:

PLANNER	- organizer
DOER	- action-oriented
MEDIATOR	- relates more to people
COMMUNICATOR	- initiates ideas

Our Personal Colouring

This finite aspect of us remains constant throughout our lives. We are either **Warm** (yellow) toned or **Cool** (blue) toned. We are either of high contrast **Colouring**, or of blended **Colouring**.

There are **Four Basic Colour Rulers**. These traits are a **Constant**, regardless of age, sex, race, or tanning. When you learn how to enhance your natural assets instead of always trying to mask them, you'll feel an incredible sense of freedom.

Colour Harmonics © A Balanced Colour system.
•   STRONG Yin – strong clear cool blue tones
•   SUBTLE Yin - soft blended cool blue tones
•   BRIGHT Yang - bright, clean warm yellow tones
•   DEEP Yang - deep, saturated warm gold tones

Our Body Shape

There are **Four Basic Body Shapes** whether short or tall. They are:

• STRAIGHT	=	Straight Narrow
• SUBSTANTIAL	=	Straight Broad
• SYMMETRICAL	=	Slight Curve
• SPHERICAL	=	Curved

Body type analysis has been under investigation since the beginning of man. Leonardo's Vitruvian man stands the test of time as the example of balance within the human body.

Even your body uses itself to determine its own balance. If you can, try this next exercise.

*Extend your arms and measure the outstretched tip to tip distance. This is your height. So, if you are looking for a long dress, use your arms minus the height of your head to ensure the right length!

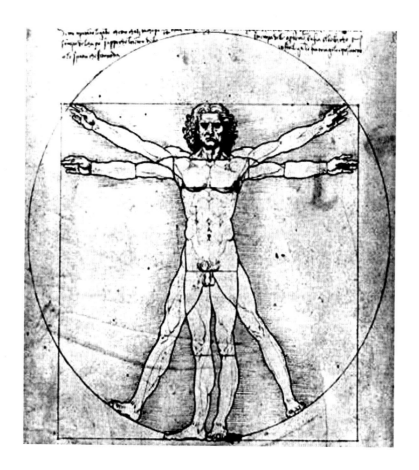

Or, when looking for a pair of shoes and don't have time to try them on? Place the shoe in the crease of your arm. Your foot fits exactly in the area between your wrist and your elbow.

If you know your own body shape measurements, it will make your shopping experiences from now on, more enjoyable, time efficient, and cost effective.

Our Style and Our Home

This corresponds directly with the other three types and again changes with age and circumstance.

Style shape terms replace the confusion induced by style terms like Contemporary, Country, Traditional, Transitional or eclectic.

The *Style Shape Terms Are*:

STRAIGHT	- planned
SUBSTANTIAL	- casual
SYMMETRICAL	- balanced
SPHERICAL	- unstructured, free form
SYNCHRONISTIC	- educated combination of styles

Discovering Your Interior Style - 8 Steps to Design Diva, combines all the above knowledge, with your personal Interior Design style. Status aside, your space should and will reveal your values. This is achieved through colours that accentuate, a style that reflects your taste, and accessories that express with confidence who occupies the space.

Each chapter or step reveals a portion of your life like a colour flower wheel. As each petal of discovery unfolds, you will become closer to the G.U.R.U. you seek.

Read, absorb and apply to reveal the real beauty you are from the inside out.

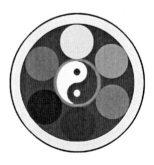

This book is about balancing your energy in all aforementioned areas to create your own unique, authentic, timeless and yet evolving image. This look and feel moves easily from personal fashion to interior design and on to your business image.

Follow these keys to find your G.U.R.U. style:

1. Spiritual - Get connected to your own higher essence and inner child.

2. Mental - Challenge your mind to recognize the box and then think outside of it.

3. Emotional - Become stable and responding rather than reactionary.

4. Physical - Become strong and healthy, while accepting and enhancing your body.

5. Financial - Obtain stability and security by saving and growing your money tree.

6. Career - Have one that inspires, creates passion and leaves a legacy.

7. Community - Give back to your home base in a way that uplifts your spirit and the neighbourhood you live in.

8. Creative Energy - Remember that even a small pebble thrown in a pond can have a ripple effect that will reach the opposite shore given the right force behind it. Make yours a positive one.

*N*otes:

Step outside yourself for a moment. Try to see yourself from a higher, less attached vantage point.

Before you even start on this discovery journey, you need to know which point of view you are coming from in order to know what, where and why you feel the need to get somewhere else.

Use the note pages at the end of each step to help clarify your thoughts. Start here with writing a sentence under each of the following categories that will help you identify your inner belief structure at a glance.

Spiritual -

Mental -

Emotional -

Physical -

Financial -

Career -

Community -

Creative Energy -

STEP 1

Discover Your Inner Traits

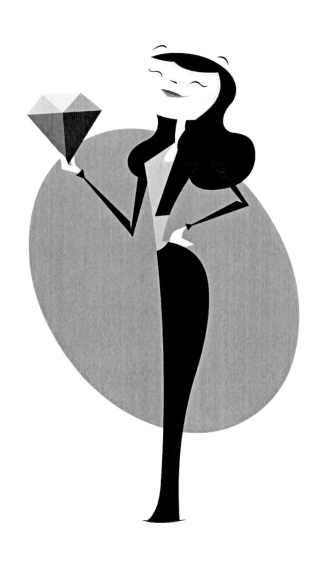

Mirror, Mirror on my desk
who's across from me
I'm trying to guess

She seems organized
but doesn't like to talk
More interested in books
then topics that are hot

The next one appears busy
always looking at her watch
She doesn't want to be here...
saw her tennis racket and socks

This lady is calm
listening with intent
weighing her words
before she comments

A flitter of laughter
comes from the one over there
Surrounded by people
laughing without a care

Mirror, Mirror on the door
It's now time to hire
one of the four

$\mathcal{S}$tep 1: Discover Your Innertraits

This is the first part of the *Infinite* side of us. Our inner character carries an essence of structure within that continues to change and evolve with education, experience and maturity.

The universe as we know it follows an expected degree of organization to function properly. We have all seen what happens when this goes awry as in hurricanes and earthquakes. We expect the sun to rise everyday giving us light and warmth and allowing us to differentiate between day and night. We look to our moon as continues it's journey non-stop around the earth pushing and pulling the tides to create our days and seasons. Not to mention how pleasantly it lights our way in the darkness of the evening.

Creatures great and small also follow an orderly arrangement. Have you ever watched ants that have discovered a honey pot? Notice how the small lookout team runs back to announce their find and within minutes a steady stream of insects arrive on the sweet scene. They have mastered the art of 'pick-up and delivery' to their lady queen who feeds and gives birth to more little troopers that will continue their lineage. OK, some would say that this structure or system isn't too bright. All one would have to do is follow the lines of ants back to their nest and poison the lot of them.

> Our inner character carries an essence of structure within that continues to change and evolve with education, experience and maturity

This reminds me of a friend of proud Scottish heritage who once described with such pride a similar scene - the military procedures of the Scottish armies of old. His eyes glazed over with a mist of reminiscence, as if he were an actual participant in that marching army.

Well, the scene played out somewhat differently in my mind. All I could see was an army that loudly announced their whereabouts to anyone within earshot. Thus, making them an easy "row upon row" target for the enemies of less regalia hiding in the trees.

Structure can be very good but, structure without knowledge and flexibility can also be very destructive. By being too focused within ourselves, our belief structures can sometimes cause us to make costly errors.

Please don't get me wrong, we need to understand and live within our structure and its limitations. But, we need to continue to evolve. This is done through education and experience to transform us into becoming well rounded human beings (I am not talking weight here!) I would liken this process to walking up a long and winding slope with many twists and turns and finally reach the top, look down and feel a renewed awareness and appreciation of the teeming meadow of life below. At that moment you realise beauty comes from four things; colour, consistency, diversity and continuous change.

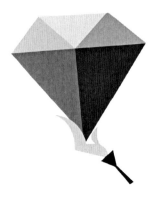

In the next few pages you will discover which of the four main innertraits is your dominant one. Once you understand your main response method you can learn to integrate all positive aspects of the other three different categories to become a true human diamond!

Your "Inner-traits"

We are all **Diamonds** in the rough! Some of us have been "through the fire," more often than others have, and have thus developed more facets to our personality. This **Infinite** area we continue to grow into. Each of us has a core or dominant personality trait but few of us are only those traits. We are usually a mixture of the four main personality categories: Planner, Doer, Mediator and/or Communicator. One of these categories is usually dominant, and the others fall in line afterwards. These categories will be discussed in detail in this chapter.

Also, understand how **You** react to others. **Four Quadrants** display this. You will react in a **Receptive** or **Reserved** manner and, you will be either **Obvious** or **Obscure** about it.

Which kind of Diamond are you?

RESERVED TYPES	RECEPTIVE TYPES
Like structure	Dislikes restrictions
Organized	Creative
Physical & mental distances from others	Prefers to deal with people rather than tasks
Work oriented	Animated, uses gestures

OBSCURE TYPES	OBVIOUS TYPES
Reserved	Fast paced
Quiet	Assertive
Co-operative	Outspoken
Supportive	Controlling
Tactful	Impatient

The sample quiz below represents a person recording their inner-traits preferences using the numbers 1 - 4. # 1 is the "least like them" and # 4 is the "most like them." You can fill in your own answers beside each question or complete the simplified version of this quiz on page 154 in Step 8.

PERSONAL:

___1___ A. I am very organized and like to have my life *planned* out so there are no surprises. I believe orderliness is next to godliness. Some people say I'm a perfectionist. I just like to pay attention to details.

___3___ B. I like to be *very productive.* I believe that idle hands make mischief, so I'm always busy. I believe a healthy body produces a healthy mind. I love sports and the outdoors.

___2___ C. I love to be in the middle of everything. *I love people, and crafts of all kinds.* I'm sensitive to others' feelings, and love to sit and chat with friends.

___4___ D. *I love peace*, and will go to almost any length to get it. Thus, I sometimes end up in the middle of problems, sorting them out, because I can usually see both sides of a situation. I'm a good listener.

FAMILY:

___1___A. I believe in family and family values. I've taught my family how to be *socially correct in all situations, and hold true to our ideals.* We are a loyal bunch that believes in doing what's right. We display a stiff upper lip when adversity comes.

___2___ B. *Our family is always on the move.* We belong to various sport groups, as well as participate in community events. My partner and I enjoy taking part in all our family's projects - that is when we have time between the two jobs that we both hold!

___3___ C. My family is playful, busy and our house is full of people all the time. We love parties, movies, and doing anything artsy and creative.

___4___ D. To me, the thought of family makes me feel warm and fuzzy like a favourite blanket. *We love to get our extended family together regularly to talk, play, or just be around each other.* We are very supportive of each other in both good times and bad.

SOCIAL:

___1___ A. *I don't really like socializing;* unless it is with a small group of *like-minded* people that share my interests and have something intelligent to offer to the conversation.

___3___ B. *My idea of socializing; is doing some sort of activity with others,* preferably sports. I love competing; it gives me a real adrenaline rush!

___2___ C. *I love parties! The more people the better.* That way, if I get bored talking to one person, I can move on to the next, and continue to enjoy the evening.

___4___ D. *I love to get together with family and friends* for a good old-fashioned meal and some sort of activity afterwards - like cards, sports, or just a good chat.

BUSINESS:

___1___ A. *I love to work with facts and figures.* Charting out profit-and-loss statements excite me. Discovering a great anomaly and writing a thesis about my findings would be great!

___2___ B. I like to be *captain of the ship. I am very result oriented.* I can accomplish more in one day, than some can in a week! I like to creatively solve problems that others are stumped by!

___3___ C. I love people, animals and anything art related! I love to tell people about new things or ideas that would really help make their life more complete. *My ideal work situation is to do anything where I can have fun, and is enjoyable for others too!*

_3_ D. *I like working with people and teaching them* how to solve their problems, be they personal, or work-related. Because I can see things from many angles, I usually end up in the middle of some trying situations.

#_4_ A's   #_10_ B's   #_10_ C's   #_16_ D's

(Dominant _D_ Secondary _B and C_)

The Grid work Key for the Diamond Character Locator is as follows: A is a Planner; B is a Doer; C is a Communicator and D is a Mediator personality type.

Using the answers filled in on the quiz: A = 4; B = 10 ; C = 10 and D = 16 As this example shows - not quite a diamond shape but getting close. The Dominant personality trait is a "D" a *Mediator* Personality type that is Receptive and Obvious about it.

There are many wonderful books and courses on personality assessment and understanding. If you have ever taken a career placement test they will have used something similar to assess which field of employment you would be most suited for and excel at.

It is about understanding your own frame of reference and skill set and then being willing to accept that others may see and do things different from you. This is where emotional detachment should come in. Unfortunately, our emotions sometimes play a bigger part than logic. We are still diamonds in the rough but diamonds none the less.

Take the test and see where you fit in the Diamond Grid.

The Diamond Character Locator

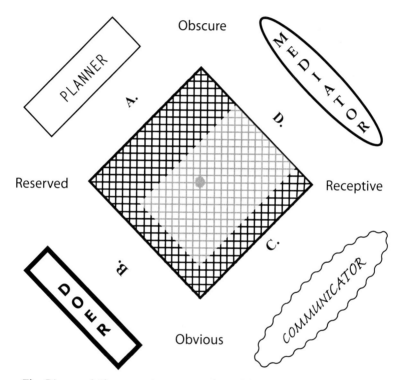

The Diamond Character Locator works as follows:

The center circle starts with a value of zero - **0**. The next line moving from the circle equals **1** - which reprepresents the *least like* **inner-trait** and **16** being the *most like* **inner-trait**. Filled in lines create the size of *diamond* you are and also illustrates your clarity or, *response* type.

If we use the answers from the quiz on pages 28 - 30 the grid would look like this: A = 4; B = 10; C = 10 and D = 16. This example shows the inner-traits of a "diamond in the rough". Close to the diamond shape we are all striving to become.

A is a **Planner**; **B** is a **Doer**; **C** is a **Communicator** and **D** is a **Mediator** personality type.

The Dominant innertrait shown is 'D', a **MEDIATOR** Personality type that is both Receptive and Obvious about it (has equal amounts of B + C.)

Here are four more questions, to reaffirm that you understand these personality types. You will find the answers to this quiz on p. 34.

1. I like to work by myself. My pace is slow and methodical. I love to handle details. Some think that I border on being a perfectionist. Who am I?

_____A. The DOER   _____B. The MEDIATOR
_____C. The PLANNER   _____D. The COMMUNICATOR

2. I don't like pushy, aggressive types. I enjoy warm, close relationships, and I am a good team player. Who am I?

_____A. The DOER   _____B. The MEDIATOR
_____C. The PLANNER   _____D. The COMMUNICATOR

3. I don't like to waste time. I enjoy challenges, taking control and solving problems. Who am I?

_____A. The DOER   _____B. The MEDIATOR
_____C. The PLANNER   _____D. The COMMUNICATOR

4. I love to be the center of attention. I like to be involved with people. I do not like to work alone, and detail work bores me to tears. I love to work with ideas, rather than data. Who am I?

_____A. The DOER   _____B. The MEDIATOR
_____C. The PLANNER   _____D. The COMMUNICATOR

After answering these questions, go to page 34 and check your answers then see how they fit with the analysis of yourself. I would venture to say that after you have completed this section, you won't look at yourself, or others in the same way.

We should all be striving to be equal in all the positive aspects of each personality category. By studying these four categories, we can then be more able to understand why each person acts and reacts differently to any given situation. Also, bear in mind that if you come across someone that really irritates you, they may be mirroring characteristics that you really dislike in yourself! Food for thought........

Use the Diamond Locator to determine how to relate to other people. If you are dealing with a Mediator, do not treat him or her like a Doer, Planner or Communicator.

Eight ways to effectively deal with each personality:

Planner

1. Be very business-like and proper.
2. Go at a slow and purposeful pace.
3. State your purpose, be it in personal or business affairs.
4. State what you plan to do.
5. Establish credibility with them.
6. Give them the facts in straight, pointed data.
7. Planners want solid, tangible proof.
8. Finally, after you have said your piece, give them space to think it over.

Be it an argument, an item to be purchased or a problem that needs solving, the most dominant question on a Planner's mind is: How does it work? The Planner's personality challenge is making timely decisions as they are constantly seeking more information.

Doer

1. Never let them see you sweat! Always walk in confidently.
2. Get to the point of your visit, chat, whatever.
3. State your purpose, by getting to the matter at hand.
4. Show consideration for their time. Doers are always busy.
5. In an argument or sales pitch, give facts, details, specifics, logical details, and your plans for all of the above - in short form.
6. Use assertive, powerful gestures to make your point (no weak hand shakes). Doers appreciate strong people.
7. Use pointed relevant humour.
8. Finally, have a contract or solution ready to be signed with a date of completion clearly visible.

Doers usually have a dry sense of humour, satirical in nature. The most dominant question that the DOER wants answered is; what you or, it can do for me by when? The Doer's Personality challenge is over committing their time, otherwise known as a do-aholic.

Mediator:

1. Reassure them that they are liked.
2. Make sure they feel that everyone is being treated fairly.
3. Offer them some guarantees.
4. Move at an easy pace, they do not like feeling pressured.
5. Listen carefully. Do not look like you would rather be somewhere else.
6. When trying to sell them on something, use third-party stories.
7. Share your feelings and opinions. They are open-minded people.
8. Before jumping into an argument, let them tell you what is important to them.

You will probably save yourself a lot of heartache. The most pressing question on the *Mediator's* mind regarding any decision is how this decision will affect me personally. Mediators need to feel safe, and know that others will not be adversely affected by their decision. The main personality challenge *Mediators* have, is the ability to **take risks**.

Communicator:

1. Walk in confidently for a chat or a business meeting.
2. Give a quick greeting.
3. Allow the *Communicator* to talk. They like nothing better than to talk about themselves, as well as what others are up to.
4. When preparing for a discussion, ask specific questions that will help guide them to the answers you need.
5. Focus your conversation on opinions and new ideas. They love to feel on top of everything happening around them.
6. Tell stories to emphasize your point. Communicators love stories.

The most pressing question on a *Communicator's* mind, whether it concerns a child's problem or sales proposition is: Who else is doing it, or who else has it? They do not like to be first in their decision making. The main personality challenge a *Communicator* has is the ability to commit to just one thing.

* ANSWERS TO THE FOUR QUESTIONS ON PAGE 33
#1 = C   #2 = B   #3 = A   #4 = D

In my forty plus years, I have come across all kinds of characters. I have learned that when you chameleon yourself into someone else's shoes a new rapport and respect can happen.

I am not saying that it will in every case. If fact, I have learned that I neither have to like or respect everyone. Nor, do they need to like or respect me back.

Whew, that was a tough one! Coming from the Mediator Personality type you just learned about, you can understand my frame of reference. Those of you of Mediator dominance know what I am talking about. Have you ever bent over backwards to help everyone you can, only to find that you have ended up ticking people off with your over zealousness and then made them feel guilty for ever asking for help. Or even worse, the objects of your help, have neither recognized, accepted or acclaimed the sacrifices you did for their benefit to the world at large. I know there are many of you all over the world suffering the same plight.

Those of Planner or Doer dominant inner traits need to ignore this rant as you have no idea what I am talking about. It is a Mediator affliction. Don't worry it isn't contagious!

The Communicator may empathize, for a moment. Wait something more exciting and pressing has capture their attention. These people are fun, and way too busy to really get depressed by your dilemma. You have to love that personality type as they help make sure you don't take yourself too seriously.

As you can see each personality type has their own frame of reference from which they react, and then respond. Understanding each type will make your social, family, & carreer life much easier.

OK, I would say that as a Mediator / Doer / Communicator personality type, I have the most trouble saying no to anyone that needs my help. Unfortunately this has gotten me into a bit of trouble from over committing myself and then having to let people down because I forgot that I was only human. It sucks! I wish that I had more time but, I am learning to accept that there are only 24 hours in each day.

It is all about balance - says the pot to the kettle....... I told you that this whole book was originally researched to the nth degree to help me understand me and the annoying little angel on my one shoulder and feisty little devil on the other.

I say grab a hat and put it on and let the hat decide who you are at that moment. I have a few hats - literally! Some are old, some new, some are character pieces. Each one brings out a different personality. No, my middle name isn't Cybil. I say try it before you knock it. In fact, I have brought out my hats, at dinner parties that were becoming decidedly too serious. When hats are donned, animation begins and laughter rules. Now, if you wear a hat for a living, try on someone elses - sort of an upside down way of "walking a mile in someone elses shoes." I think that the only way we can have a total human experience is by breaking bread with people that are opposite to you in outlook, colour, and career and put on a silly hat. Somehow that makes everyone equal and the differences diminish.

> Life is really about giving and having love, a home, friends, respect and a sense of humour.

Life is really about giving and having love, a home, friends, respect and a sense of humour. That and have a pet. They still love you even when you are at your worst, empathize with you when you are down and cheer you up with their crazy antics. Yes truly, pets and hats are the secret to a full life.

Now that you have an idea of your own personality type and traits it will be simple and fun to access and understand others better. This is the beginning of easy communication and cooperation.

All of us inhabiting this earth want basically the same 8 things:

1. A loyal and loving family.

2. A warm place to sleep and call home.

3. Good food on the table with positive conversation and laughter.

4. Helpful and supportive friends.

5. A fulfilling job or career.

6. Respect.

7. Acceptance and appreciation, and finally

8. A sense of purpose for why we are here.

Once those issues have been looked after, we can then begin to feather our nests. This is where I have fun! In the next book - *Discovering Your Interior Style - 8 Steps to Design Diva*, I look forward to helping you create the living space of your dreams easily and affordably!

*N*otes:

Use this page as a thinking page and create your own diamond traits picture. After you are finished you can transfer the information on your own personalized diamond grid in Step 8 page 155.

STEP 2

*W*ear Your Power Colours

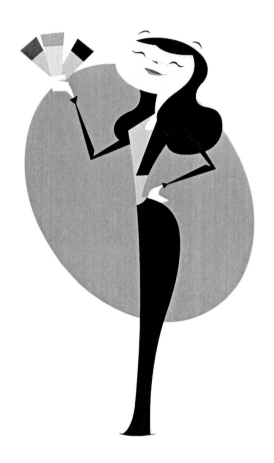

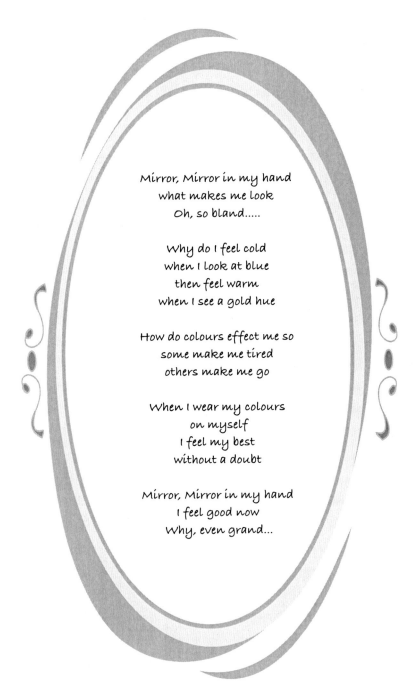

Mirror, Mirror in my hand
what makes me look
Oh, so bland.....

Why do I feel cold
when I look at blue
then feel warm
when I see a gold hue

How do colours effect me so
some make me tired
others make me go

When I wear my colours
on myself
I feel my best
without a doubt

Mirror, Mirror in my hand
I feel good now
Why, even grand...

$\mathcal{S}$tep 2: Wear Your Power Colours

COLOUR HARMONICS® The colour ruler system

Before we delve into personal colour, we need to learn a little history about this subject that affects us all - colour

Why do we buy items that contain colour? Is it because colour fills a need within us? Just think, if we didn't, all our belongings would look like we just got them out of a tapioca pudding box.

Have you ever thought about how colour affects you? Even our language expresses colour.
- *I am feeling blue.*
- *I am in the red again.*
- *That makes me green with envy, etc.*

Have you ever walked into an all blue room and felt cool and then walked into a terra cotta coloured room in the same house and felt warm? Why?

Did you know that colour radiates energy? In fact, science has proven that everything radiates energy! Most of these emanations are invisible to the naked eye (a trained eye can see them). Instruments like the thermograph, detects body heat. Do you remember the old movie *Total Recall* with Arnold Schwarzenegger? They used this technology to show the movements of people through buildings.

Many different colour theories are used today. I have condensed this information and will deal with the most commonly asked questions later in this chapter.

The History Of Colour

Colour theories go back more than two thousand years, there has been, and continues to be, a wealth of wonderful work contributing to our understanding of colour. Colour is one of life's greatest mysteries. There has never been a time when colour did not fascinate humanity. (If you find colour as fascinating as I do, go to the index at the back of this book for some websites and books on this wonderful subject.)

A Quick Colour History Lesson

In the fourth century BC, the great philosopher, Aristotle, considered blue and yellow to be the true primary colours, relating as they do to life's polarities: sun and moon, male and female, stimulus and sedation, expansion and contraction, out and in. Furthermore, he associated colours with the four elements: fire, water, earth and air. (Sounds like *Yin* and *Yang* to me!)

> The greatest contributions to our understanding of colour came from men whose work combined science and mathematics with art, metaphysics and theology.

Hippocrates, the father of medical practice, a contemporary of Aristotle used colour extensively in medicine and recognized the therapeutic effects of a white violet would be quite different from those of a purple (violet) one. The greatest contributions to our understanding of colour came from men whose work combined science and mathematics with art, metaphysics and theology. Unfortunately, by the latter part of the nineteenth century, the medical community had virtually all but erased the age-old practice of colour therapy, dismissing it as "mumbo-jumbo".

Thankfully now in the twentieth and twenty-first century the interest in colour has exploded. The art of colour therapy has been re-born and today some of the most mainstream doctors use colour as an everyday part of their work.

In the 1920s at the famous Bauhaus school, in Germany, where the teaching staff included such luminaries as Itten, Albers, Kandinsky, Mondrian and Klee, technology and art were completely reunited. Johannes Itten was particularly interested in the connections between colours and emotions, and colours and shapes. He also observed that each of his students seemed to favour the same palette for their work - and furthermore, the favoured palette appeared to be in some way related to that student's own physical colouring. Itten's seminal book, "The Art of Colour," is a "must read" for anyone interested in colour.

> For centuries, colours were thought to be part of the object viewed.

The Science Behind Colour

Where does colour come from? For centuries, colours were thought to be part of the object viewed. In 1672, the great scientist, Sir Isaac Newton, published his first controversial paper on colour and forty years later, his work Opticks. When Newton shone white light through a triangular prism, he found that wavelengths of light refracted at different angles, enabling him to see the separate components – colours.

In 1840, Johannes Wolfgang von Goethe's, Theory of Colours disputed Newton's prism experiments and proved that light splits into its component colours. He himself shone white light on to a screen in a room and found that the centre of the image remained white and colours appeared only at the edges. This led him back to Aristotle's ideas that blue is the first colour to appear out of darkness (and most visible at night) and yellow is the first colour to appear out of light (and the most visible colour in light conditions). Therefore, our perception of the sun is that we are looking at white light as being yellow and the vast blackness of space as appearing blue.

When a white beam of light is shot through a prism it registers all the visible colours of the electromagnetic spectrum from red to violet.

Of the tiny portion we see as visible light, Red has the longest wavelength – closest to black light (absorption of all colours) and Violet has the shortest wavelength - closest to white light (reflection of all colours). All other colours fall somewhere in between.

Colour Therapists often refer to these pure colours as "rays."

The sun is our local source of almost all the electromagnetic spectrum both long and short waves. Our atmosphere screens out most of the harmful rays so when we damage our atmosphere by pollution, we ultimately hurt ourselves.

> Each colour of the spectrum moves to a different wavelength.

So, round and round we go and come back to the theory that the origin of colour is light. Without light, we would not be able to distinguish the differences between colours. Light travels in waves. The wave is a characteristic movement of all types of energy. Light is a small portion of the electromagnetic spectrum, which also includes X-rays, ultraviolet and infrared light, microwaves and radio waves. Each colour of the spectrum moves to a different wavelength. Colour is magic and can even appear to play games with our mind.Some of the most common tricks are as follows:

Colour Illusions and Effects

Afterimage: This image is related to simultaneous contrast.Simply stated, if you stare at one colour long enough and close your eyes, you'll see its complementary colour; eg., red creates a green afterimage.

Light on texture and finishes: Basically the same colour can be applied to several surfaces, and all appear different due to the inherent distinctions of the surface used.

Metamerism: Using a colorimeter will show that some colours don't have the same reflectance curve. They can appear to match under certain lights, but not under others.

Simultaneous contrast: This colour phenomenon was discovered by Michael Eugene Chevreul.He discovered that each hue projects its complement on the adjacent hue.Therefore, to receive the maximum intensity of a hue, surround it with its complement!

Value Relationships: Degree of the lightness or darkness of a colour is affected by the adjacent colour values.Strong contrasts cause light areas to appear lighter and dark areas to appear darker.

Natural light: even in natural daylight, there are differences seen in colour.

- Late evening to early morning starts the cool end of the spectrum, intense in colour and contrast (Strong Yin).By late morning to early afternoon clear and sunny yellow (Bright Yang) infuse all colours.

- The afternoon carries a softer tone to the colours, with medium intensity due to the diffusion of light by the sun.(Subtle Yin)

- By evening, the colours that surround us have a deep saturation that tends to the warm end of the spectrum. (Deep Yang)

The Inner Psychology Behind Colours

Colour evokes feelings. These feelings have come from many sources, like fond memories or traumatic events; maybe they are associated with cultural, ethnic or religious beliefs. It is important to understand your underlying view of the colours you have chosen for personal, home or business use. Following are some ideas of how colour may unconsciously effect us:

WHITE	Yang	Colour

Physical: - White light contains all colours and is the reflection of all colours

Emotional: - Represents revelation –"I've been enlightened", innocence and radiance

Mental: Represents the positive, purity, masculine, active force, *Yang*

Negative Aspect: Too much power, even positive, can destroy instead of create if it is not balanced

BLACK | Yin | Colour

Physical: Absence of all light, or negation of all colour, the absorption of all colours

Emotional: Represents the physical, material, or earthy (Mother Earth)

Mental: Represents the negative (not evil), feminine, receptive form, *Yin*

Negative Aspect: Seen as evil, dark, mourning (Western belief) or black magic

BROWN | Ying | Colour

Physical: Brown usually consists of green, red and yellow, and a large percentage of black

Emotional: Much of the same seriousness as black, but warmer and softer. It has associations with the earth and the natural world

Mental: It is a solid, reliable colour and most people find it quietly supportive

Negative Aspect: Lack of humour, heaviness, lack of sophistication

GRAY | Ying | Colour

Physical: Combination of Black/ White and possibly Brown

Emotional: Psychological neutrality. Heavy use of grey usually indicates a lack of confidence and fear of exposure

Mental: Suppressive as absence of colour is depressing

Negative Aspect: Lack of confidence, dampness, depression, lack of energy, hibernation.

RED | Yang | Primary Colour - longest wavelength

Physical: Revitalizing effect on our bodies, clears impurities from the blood stream, vital energy

Emotional: Intensity of feeling, achievement, ambition, "grounding to earth"

Mental: Initiator, creator, the pioneer colour

Negative Aspect: Too much red can result in agitation, (from anger to destruction). Use as an accent to enliven and create warmth

PINK | Yin | Tint of Red

Physical: It soothes, rather than stimulates

Emotional: Represents the feminine principle and survival of the species; to sooth, nurture, create warmth, femininity, love, sexuality

Mental: Powerful colour. Too much pink is physically draining and can be somewhat emasculating.

Negative: Inhibition, emotional claustrophobia, emasculation, physical weakness

ORANGE | Yang | Secondary Colour (Red + Yellow)

Physical: Body cleanser, an aid to colds, digestion & asthma.

Emotional: Buoyant colour that can lift the spirits – warm peaceful colour that allows freedom of expression and creativity

Mental: Self-motivation allows for ambition and change, a rebirth so to speak

Negative Aspect: If tone is towards the red end of the scale, in large amounts, it can become an aggressive colour. If tone is towards the yellow end, in large amounts, it can become domineering

YELLOW | Yang | Primary Colour

Physical: Has a stimulating and refreshing quality about it. It helps with indigestion and restoring tattered nerves – use to brighten up an otherwise dark, or cool room

Emotional: Yellow personality is always compulsively looking at the future in child-like anticipation

Mental: Awakens the intellect, good to use in a child's study room.

Negative Aspect: If used in large amounts, can appear overpowering; uncultured and child-like, seeking isolation and protection from disappointment

GREEN | Ying | Secondary Colour - Blue + Yellow

Physical: Helps to reduce high blood pressure, beneficial to the nervous system, a colour that promotes peace and harmony in any environment

Emotional: The Balance Colour of new life and growth that requires the reason behind belief systems

Mental: A very practical, self-assertive, transitional colour used by all personality types

Negative Aspect: Personified- if green does not receive due recognition, tension and distress, leading to jealousy and envy, can take over control. Balance is the key

BLUE | Yin | Primary Colour - short wavelength

Physical: Helps to heal the mind / brain, and all components. Also cools the blood, to relieve swollen conditions

Emotional: Peaceful, relaxing, and soothing

Mental: Think sky, oceans, space. A very expansive colour that is peaceful and harmonious

Negative Aspect: Personified- if used exclusively, tends to become cold and unfeeling, creating a sense of melancholy, and a life that does not measure up to one's ideals

INDIGO | Yin | Tertiary Colour - Blue + Violet

Physical: Here is a helpful colour for the insomniacs, or those with eye, ear, or nose problems. In homes or clothes, use as a background colour.

Emotional: A calming colour that helps dispel the feeling of frustration and negativity associated with mental conflict

Mental: An uplifting, artistic and spiritual colour; cool and mysterious, that is becoming more popular today

Negative Aspect: An indigo personality can become conceited or full of contempt for those that do not understand them and their work

VIOLET | Ying | Secondary Colour - Blue + Red

Physical: Helps to stimulate the electrochemical elements of the nerves, creating a cool, tonic-like effect for the whole body

Emotional: A mysterious colour that seems to permeate reality with vision

Mental: Is the combination of a spiritual blue and realistic, artistic indigo

Negative Aspect: Violet personalities can appear to be critical and obsessed with injustice, but unwilling to change the situation.

The Four Colour Harmonic© Rulers

In this next section, we will actually discover your particular **Colour Harmonics**© Colour Ruler. If you have been colour-coded in the past, this will prove to be an interesting twist. If not, you will need to get a few items before we begin.

- Full daylight spectrum light (or natural daylight)
- Mirror (large enough to see your head and shoulders)
- Gold metallic cloth and a silver metallic cloth
- Colour Harmonic Characteristic sheets

Match the colours below to the swatches in Step 8 to make a fabric drape:

- Jet-black cloth	- Pantone # Black 6
- Wheat cloth	- Pantone # 466
- Rootbeer	- Pantone # 478
- Mauve taupe	- Pantone # 437

*NOTE: All fabrics should be a minimum of 18" x 36", to cover the upper body. To create the most accurate personal colouring results, you should wear a white or, very neutral coloured head wrap and robe to prevent possible distraction from unnatural hair dye or clothing colours. I also recommend wearing a white or neutral robe. You must also remove all make-up, or the test will be invalid.

One of the first decisions you make each day involves colour harmony. "What am I going to wear?" Whether you're choosing clothing, make-up or designing a new room, the colours you choose affect your final results.

Colour is light and light is energy. As you just learned, scientists have found that mental and physical changes take place when you're exposed to colours. They can stimulate, excite, depress, tranquillize, and create a feeling of well-being and peace.

The Colour Harmonic Ruler

Let me introduce to you *Colour Harmonics* © - the colour ruler system. Several convenient and easy-to-use tools in Step 8 will assist you in making the best colour decision whenever you purchase clothing, accessories and make-up. These tools also are made to help you purchase items for your home environment i.e. paint, wallpaper, furniture and fabrics. Now you can take control of how you communicate and live with colour.

Here's how the system works:

Each of the four Colour Harmonic© groups will be described in detail this chapter. I have selected colours, arranged in four ways: in Step 8, four mini rulers are displayed. Two of these rulers illustrate the cool, blue tones of the *Yin* colour side and the other two display the warm, yellow under-toned or *Yang* colour side.

Each Colour Harmonic tool (hereafter referred to as CH) is bordered on the top and bottom by its metallic compliment. Gold is used for warm rulers (Bright and Deep Yang) and silver is used for the cool rulers (Strong and Subtle Yin). Here are the basic differences:

• While both Bright and Deep Yang are considered warm colours, but they differ in their intensity. Bright Yang has clear, bright colours with a soft yellow undertone and Deep Yang has saturated and muted colours with a golden undertone.

• Strong and Subtle Yin colours are cool, but Strong Yin contains pure, intense, and high saturated blue based colours and Subtle Yin contains more grayed, blended and soft pastel blue based tones CH also has three power neutrals on the top portion, and is followed by 9 harmonized accent colours. Neutrals are the staples that you build a wardrobe or interior around. These are background colours that can be used in large amounts. Accents blend with the neutrals and introduce a punch of colour to give them life.

On page 60 the CH Ying colour flower is introduced. You can see the colour version of the Colour Harmonic© Tool in the colour insert, after page 159. Each colour group is also introduced with its harmonious colour collage.

View the following items in the full colour section after page 159:
- Four pantone colours used for assessing your colour group
- Four Yin & Yang Mini Colour Rulers
- Four CH colour Collages
- Four Make-up style examples

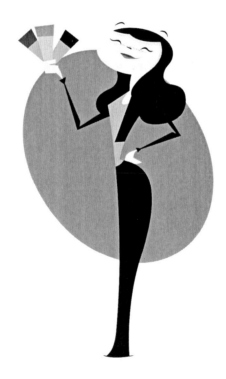

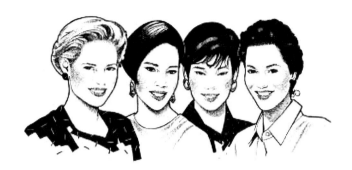

Under normal circumstances, skin colour and tone remains constant throughout our lives. These colours can change somewhat, due to the following factors: diet change, (too much carrot juice), medical problems, jaundice, anaesthetic during surgery, skin grafting or plastic surgery can also alter the outward appearance of the skin. Nevertheless, understand that the basic undertone and composition of our skin remains constant.

In this book, we will be concerned about colour harmonies. These are the colours that enhance our skin, hair and eyes. Healthy, natural hair colour is automatically coordinated with the colour of our complexion and eyes. Even during the aging process (as those components change) coordination and harmony remains.

We are the artist or creator of our own image. As such, we should be trying to make a life-size picture of harmony. This is where cosmetics can play an important part (lipstick, blush, foundation, and any other cosmetics used). When we use cosmetic colours that blend with our natural colouring, then the overall appearance is pleasing. If colours are used, that are in discord with the skin and hair, the overall effect is not as pleasing to the eye. An example of this is: a dark brunette, with brown eyes and olive skin, dyes his/her hair a bleached platinum blond - a definite discord is seen. Likewise, if a redhead, with peach skin and freckles, dyes his/her hair jet black, discord is very evident. Whether you are a blonde, black, brown or red haired person if enhanced correctly your inner person will shine through.

All colours, even neutrals, have a warm or cool undertone. when you wear your "power neutral colours" they act as the base that supports and balances your skin colour to your clothes and environment.

Once you have confirmed whether you are warm-toned, (gold cloth), or cool-toned, (silver cloth), try the other four cloths to confirm your findings. Look at the area around your nose and mouth. Do you see shadows and little lines that you did not even realize were there? On the other hand, does your complexion look smooth and youthful, with a rested, rather than tired look? The former is not in harmony with your natural colouring, and the latter is.

> Incorporate your power neutral colours and they will act as the base that supports and balances your skin colour to your clothes and environment.

The reason I have selected the following four colours, is that only those with a particular skin tone will look good in the chosen colour.

Jet Black Cloth	=	**Strong Yin**
Mauve Taupe	=	**Subtle Yin**
Wheat Yellow	=	**Bright Yang**
Rootbeer Brown	=	**Deep Yang**

If You're Deciding Between Colour Rulers Ask Yourself:

Strong Vs Deep:
Am I better in black, pure white, clear colours = (Strong Yin); or brown, pumpkin and muted gold = (Deep Yang)? Brown is boring on a Strong Yin, but is exciting on a Deep Yang.

Strong Vs Subtle:
Do I look good in pastels like powder pink or blue = (Subtle); or do I need darker or brighter colours, because pastels make me look washed out = (Strong) ?

Strong Vs Bright: Am I really terrific in ivory, yellow and bright navy = (Bright); or better in black, pure white and dark colours = (Strong)?

Subtle Vs Deep: Am I great in pastel blues, blue greens and pinks, but not good in pumpkin or mustard colours (Subtle), or vice versa (Deep)?

Deep Vs Bright: Do I wear muted colours like mustard and moss green, or very dark brown (Deep Yang), or am I better in clear colours like buff, light clear gold, peach and lighter golden browns (Bright Yang)? Neither right? - Try Subtle!

Once you have determined which Colour Harmonic Ruler you belong to, the next step is to find out which of those colours enhance our natural colouring.

Here are answers to some frequently asked questions:

Q. I have heard that having your "Colours" done is coming back in Vogue, is this true? Why is this important? Also, I had my colours done years ago and I do not like or wear the colours selected for me, why?

A. Yes, personal Colour Consultation is back. Actually it never left. It is a tool largely used by Image Consultants to help their clients with their clothing, make-up and hair colour selections. As far as not liking the colours selected for yourself, a couple of things may have been at fault. One, errors have occurred in colour identification because some Colour Consultants weren't trained properly and /or had the skill level to identify the undertones of colour in different individuals. Secondly, due to the increased diversification of personal care and fashion products, re-education and experimentation, personal colour theories have adapted and changed. For example: you can now use a blend of warm and cool neutral products to balance your colouring and create a more approachable look and/or environment. (Help from a Colour or Image Consultant to accomplish this is advised.)

Q. Can I be a mixture of *Colour Harmonies*?

A. Yes, it is genetically possible. If your parents or grandparents are of mixed races, it is possible. For example if your mother is Scandinavian and your father is Japanese there is a good chance that you will have a mixture of colouration in your skin. One undertone (warm or cool) however will always be dominant.

Q. Can I be a mixture of *Colour Intensities*?

A. It is possible but not the norm. The basic law of abstract colour theory states that the base of a colour determines its shade. Your skin tone is the same. Olive skin has a blue undertone. High contrast *Colouring* needs clear shades, to enhance and bring out the intensity. Blended *Colouring* needs saturated colours, to allow the subtlety of your colour to show through. If you mix dusty tones with clear, it only negates your particular *Colouring* group. In make-up especially, all colours should be in one colour family but balanced by use of the opposite neutral to soften the contrast if your skin has a mixture of colour intensity.

Note: Personal colouring characteristics for descendants of North American Indians, Africans, Asians, and Latin Americans:

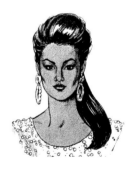

Persons, who have inherited their *Colouring* from one of the above races, are most often *Strong Yin* in colouring. However, some will be found in each of the other groups

Skin tone is the main determining factor, since hair colour can be black in all groups.

Cool "Yin" Colour Groups: Strong And Subtle
The range of skin tones include white or ivory, olive, beige, rose beige, rose brown, ash brown, red brown, dark brown and blue black. When compared to the *Strong*, the *Subtle's* skin tone is either lighter, more grayed, or rosy. The *Subtle's* eyes are not as dark. There is a softer, more muted look to the skin and eyes, rather than black. The hair may be ash brown, or dark brown.

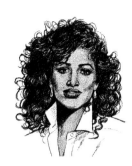

Warm "Yang" Colour Groups:
Bright & Deep

The range of skin tones includes ivory, peach, beige, golden beige, copper, bronze, caramel and golden brown, (light to dark). Skin tone must be a true golden, not olive green colour. Eyes will be dark brown, not black, or golden brown or even hazel. Hair might still be black, but may also be dark brown, with some gold, chestnut, or red in it. Sometimes, there may even be a light, golden-brown tone in it.

Intuitively sense - your Colour Harmonic's *Group is*:

_____

Skin Colour: _____

Eye Colour: _____

Natural Hair Colour: _____

Blended Colouring: _____

High Contrast Colouring : _____

Final Analysis of your Colour Group: _____

Points To Remember For Each Colour Ruler

Bright: Has a clear yellow undertone to skin. Use all five hues of colour with yellow added. Use bright, clear colours. High Contrast between hair, skin and eyes

Deep: Has warm golden undertone to skin. Use all five hues of colour with golden yellow added. Use rich, mellow colours. Blended Colouring between hair, skin and eyes

Subtle: Has soft blue undertone to skin. Use all five hues of colour with blue added. Use soft, pastel colours. Blended Colouring between hair, skin and eyes

Strong: Has cool blue undertone to skin. Use all five hues of colour with blue added, as well as primary colours. Clear, blue, and vivid colours look best. High Contrast between hair, skin and eyes

Time to Discover Your Power Colours!

Do you have all the necessary items needed? Make-up removed? Head wrap on? Now shine the lamp on your face and you're ready to proceed. This works really well with a friend that can be very objective.

OK, face the mirror and begin by draping the gold, then silver cloth around your face. Which colour brings your face to life? You don't want to blend into the colour like a cool-toned person will, if they put the gold cloth next to them. This is especially true of a *Strong* - coloured individual. Their face will appear yellow and sickly.

Look at the areas around the mouth, and around the eyes. If your eyes look tired and rather listless, this colour is in disharmony with your natural colouring. If your eyes look bright and shiny and even more their colour, this colour is in harmony with your **natural** Colouring.

As stated in the introduction, what we are trying to achieve in this book, is balance and harmony, not exact specifics and scientific dogma.

This is an overview, allowing each of the subjects to intertwine together, instead of being treated as separate entities. Each subject is truly a book, in and of itself. I hope that this information spurs you on to a more in-depth study of whichever subject fascinates you. My purpose is to give those with a lot of curiosity, but little time, a place to find some much needed answers, in a simple format.

Now that we have a few of the most commonly asked questions out of the way, let us begin by understanding how Personal *Colouring* works.

There are four identifiable groups.

Warm Tones:
　　Bright Yang - think bright sunlit colours
　　Deep Yang - think deep golden sunsets

Cool Tones:
　　Strong Yin - think of a full moon at midnight
　　Subtle Yin - think of the cool softness of dusk.

Read the *Colouring* characteristic pages following for each group. Go through each section and mentally mark off those characteristics that most describe you and transfer this information to your personal colouring sheet on page 164.

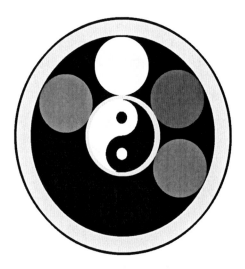

Each *Ying* flower is unique to its colour harmonic's group.

The background displays the strongest power neutral.
The Yin/Yang symbol in the centre the light and dark neutral.

Each petal starts with its version of yellow at the top and moves around like a colour wheel replacing each petal with it's colour base corrected tone.

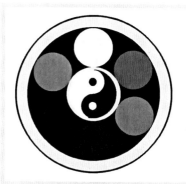

STRONG:

YIN

- Intense, Blue Based Colours

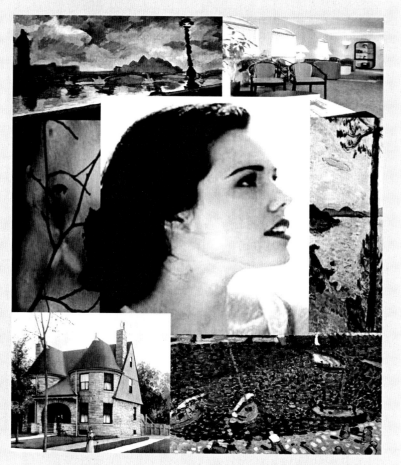

Strong Yin

True primary colours - with blue added to them. Whether true or blue they are clear & vibrant.

Cosmetics

Strong's can apply more dramatic make-up than other seasons, but lighter make-up is also flattering.

Foundation: Pink or rose base. Avoid yellow/orange.

Lipstick/nail Colour: Deep, strong rose or pink, plum, burgundy, true red, blue/red. Clear colours, not muted.

Blusher: Pink, plum, red.

Eye Shadow: Smoked or silvery blues, gray, mauve, or plum. If colour is too bright, add gray or a taupe brown to soften the colour.

Hair Colour: A *Strong* should keep their colour as long as possible. A good colourist can add the right tone of highlights so as not to negate your striking colouring. Think rich mahogany or jet black accents that look quite striking as well as salt and pepper to pure white as we age.

Accessories

Shoes & Handbags: Black, navy, grey, burgundy, taupe, bone, white, silver.

Hosiery: Gray-beige, and tones of your palette.

Glasses: Silver, gunmetal, black or rich coloured frames that coordinate with your palette. Two tone Black / Brown or Silver and gold are good.

Jewelry: Smooth or shiny, simple or heavily detailed. Match your jewelry to your personal style. ie: Exotic, Natural, Classic or Romantic.

Metals: White-gold, platinum, silver or mixed metals like silver and gold.

Gems: White and black pearls, emeralds, rubies, sapphires, jade, jet crystal. Clear, sparkling stones are best. Especially diamonds!

Strong Yin Colouring

A Strong has high contrast between their hair, eyes and skin colours. A typical Strong has dark hair and eyes with a much lighter skin tone by comparison.

Colours To Wear

Reds: Poinsettia red, scarlet, rich blue-reds, burgundy. No orange-red.

Blue: Deep blues, royal blues, blue-purple, any navy, electric blue, bright turquoise.

Yellow: Only butter yellow, No gold, no orange.

Green: Emerald green, deep blue-greens, No yellow-greens .

Purple: Purple blues, royal purple, rich, deep purple.

Brown: If you wear brown, it should be a black / brown or charcoal brown, worn with black accessories. No other browns. The only beige, is taupe (greyed beige).

Icy Tones: Very pale, icy versions of your colours are especially effective in a fabric that has a texture that glows or shimmers. No pastels.

Black & White: Midnight black and stark white to tooth white. True gray.

Good Basic Colours: Pure white, soft true gray, charcoal gray, black, navy, taupe, burgundy. Intense deep vivid colours are magnificent on a Strong Yin. Colours should be clear and pure, not muted or powdered. If lighter tints are used, they should be cool, icy values of colour.

Strong's don't wear middle value colours well. Dark /light colour contrasts, or monochromatic colour schemes, are very effective and just as striking as complimentary colour combinations. Solid colours are best, but high-contrast prints work as well.

A Strong Yin's Basic Colour Wardrobe

Work Wear:	Winter	Summer
Jacket	Black	White
Skirt	Gray	White
Pants	Black	Navy
Dress	Red	True Green
Blouse 1	Icy Gray	True Red
Blouse 2	Purple/Red/Black Print	Navy/White
Dressy Blouse	White	Purple
Sweater	Magenta	Navy (Knit)
Cocktail Pants	Black	White
Skirt Or Dress	Black	White

Casual Wear:	Winter	Summer
Casual Pants	Navy	White
Casual Skirt	Navy	White
Casual Top	Red	Magenta
Coat	Black	White
Trench Coat	Taupe (Grey-beige)	Icy Gray
Evening Wrap	Emerald Green	White Shawl

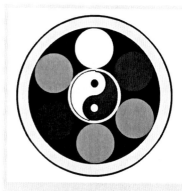

SUBTLE:

YIN

- Muted Blue Tones

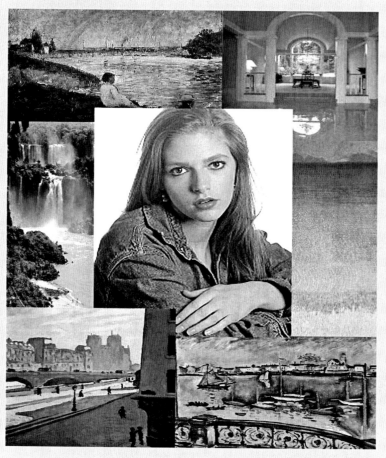

Subtle Yin

Subtles Five Basic Hues (Primary) with blue added. Colours are best when blended or dusty.

Cosmetics

Subtles should try and create a soft, blended look in their make-up. Strong, or dark colours, will make them appear harsh.

Foundation: Pink/ rose beige. Avoid yellow/tan base.

Lipstick/nail Colour: Pink, rose, mauve, soft burgundy.

Blusher: Pink, rose, plum.

Eye Shadow: Violet or lavender, blues, blue-green. Greyed or smoky tones. Avoid overly dramatic eye make-up. Go for the blended look, and add gray or taupe brown if the colour is too bright.

Hair Colour: Soft delicate shades with ash tones, no gold or red. Frosting is good for highlights, and wonderful effects can be achieved with ash blond tints on greying hair. Silver hair can be glamorous on a *Subtle*.

Accessories

Shoes And Handbags: Gray, blue-gray, soft navy, rose-brown, bone, silver.

Hosiery: Rose or gray-beige and tones of your palette.

Glasses: Frames in a nickel or silver metal, or soft tones of your palette that coordinates with most of your colours.

Jewelry: Silver toned, pewter, white gold or platinum, and any colour that blends with your colours, soft and muted.

Gems: Stones that glow, rather than sparkle. Opal, star sapphire, pink and blue sapphire, amethyst, cameos, ivory and rose ivory, moonstone, pink coral, pink pearls.

Subtles wear pearls better than any other Colour Harmonics Colour Group.

Subtle Yin Colouring

A Subtle's colouring is more translucent than a Strong's colouring as they have more rosy tones appearing at the surface of their skin.

They look best when they use softer and more dusty blue undertone colours in their makeup and hair.

Subtle colours are harmonious in their muted hues, tinged with rose or blue, often greyed like the soft incandescence of twilight. Shades are soft, not intense, as though seen through a gentle haze.

Good Basic Colours: Soft white, blue-grays, silver-grays, rose-beige, dusty rose, greyed navy.

Colours To Wear

Red: Blue tones, not too dark. Soft wine tones. No orange-red.

Pink: Blue base pastel to deep rose. Not peach

Blue: Most blues, from pale to medium. Periwinkle blue gray. Navy.

Violet: Lilac and lavender. Deeper violet pinks.

Yellow: Only pale butter yellow. Not gold or orange.

Green: Pale to medium blue-green. Pale aqua. Not yellow green.

Grey: Tones of silver and blue-grey.

Brown: Pale rose-brown, or greyed, soft brown.

White: Soft white (hint of grey or beige, no yellow).

A Subtle Yin's Basic Colour Wardrobe

Work Wear:	Winter	Summer
Jacket	Blue-gray	Soft
White Skirt	Blue-gray	Soft White
Pants	Slate Blue	Grayed Navy
Dress	Raspberry	Sky Blue
Blouse 1	Soft Wine	Blue-green
Blouse 2	PlumRose	Off White Print
Dressy Blouse	Soft White	Grayed Navy
Sweater	Soft Blue-red	Grayed Navy
Cocktail Pants	Burgundy	Pale - Rose Brown
Skirt Or Dress	Burgundy	Pale - Rose Brown

Casual Wear:	Winter	Summer
Casual Pants	Cocoa	Gray - Blue
Casual Skirt	Cocoa	Gray - Blue
Casual Top	Blue - Green	Watermelon
Coat	Grayed Navy	Soft White
Trench Coat	Rose Beige	Powder Blue
Evening Wrap	Burgundy	Soft White

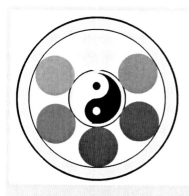

BRIGHT:

YANG

- Clear Golden Colours

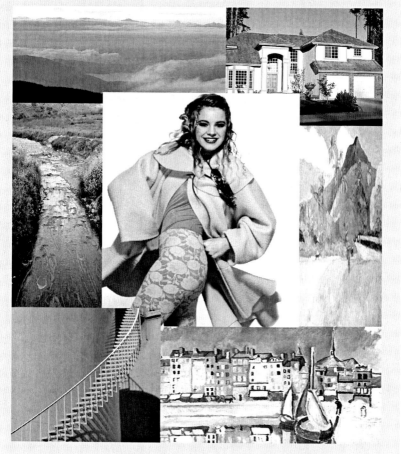

Bright Yang

Five basic hues with yellow added. Colours are clear, & best in shades lighter in value.

Cosmetics

Bright's should have very light-looking make-up.

Foundation: Yellow-based beige, ivory or peach. Avoid pink tones.

Lipstick/nail Colour: Peach, apricot, coral, warm pink, clear orange/red. Avoid browns. Use clear tones, not too dark.

Blusher: Peach or apricot, warm pink.

Eye shadow: Yellow-green, turquoise, aqua, peach, golden brown. Keep eye shadow subtle and iridescent. Add warm brown, if too bright.

Hair Colour: Try to have glistening hair - avoid a dull look. Keep gray out of your hair as long as possible. Tint your hair with golden blonde, golden brown; or red, if you are a redhead.

Accessories

Shoes And Handbags: Tan, golden brown, camel, light navy, ivory, gold.

Hosiery: Golden beige, and tones of your palette.

Glasses: Gold metal frames, or pale tones of your palette that coordinates with your colours.

Jewelry: Gold metal, or any bright or light tones from your palette. Use a pale yellow gold to pick up hair and skin highlights. Bronze or copper is usually overpowering. Green gold is good.

Gems: Creamy pearls, coral, opals, yellow topaz, turquoise, aquamarine, yellow sapphire. Try to use stones that sparkle.

Bright Yang Colouring

Bright's have clear and bright eyes and complexion. They have a high contrast between their eyes, hair and skin but with a clear yellowish undertone that appears peach like instead of pink.

The colours of a *Bright* are alive with sunlight, radiant and fresh. Colour clarity is the main thing to consider. They can be vivid or delicate, but not muted or dark. Although Bright's have a delicate quality, they are the most radiant and eternally youthful of all the colour groups.

Colours To Wear

Red: Orange or yellow reds. No blue-reds, no burgundy.

Pink: Peach or coral pinks. No blue-pink.

Blue: Bright blue, clear navy, periwinkle blue, peacock, turquoise.

Violet: Medium tone, warm violets.

Yellow: Soft daffodil yellow, sand, clear golden yellow.

Green: Yellow-greens, lime, pale or bright, aqua.

Gray: Soft yellow-gray.

Brown: Beige, camel. Golden - honey browns, not too dark. No rose-browns. Light rust.

White: Creamy ivory.

Orange: Light clear tints, apricot.

Black: Can wear a golden Khaki black not a strong blue black

Good Basic Colours: Ivory, sand, beige, camel, golden browns, warm gray, clear navy, peach.

A Bright Yang's Basic Colour Wardrobe

Work Wear:	Winter	Summer
Jacket	Clear Navy	Ivory
Skirt	Clear Navy	Ivory
Pants	Camel	Clear Navy
Dress	Tomato Red	Peach
Blouse 1	Clear Salmon	Light Periwinkle
Blouse 2	Orange-Red	Bright Coral
Dressy Blouse	Lt. Warm Beige	Kelly Green
Sweater	Camel	Clear Navy
Cocktail Pants	Lt. Warm Beige	Ivory
Skirt Or Dress	Lt. Warm Beige	Ivory

Casual Wear:	Winter	Summer
Casual Pants	Golden Tan	Wheat
Casual Skirt	Golden Tan	Wheat
Casual Top	Periwinkle	Light Clear Gold
Coat	Golden Brown	Light Warm Beige
Trench Coat	Lt. Warm Beige	Ivory
Evening Wrap	Ivory	Soft White

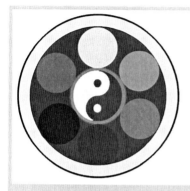

Deep:

Yang

- Rich, Saturated Golden Tones

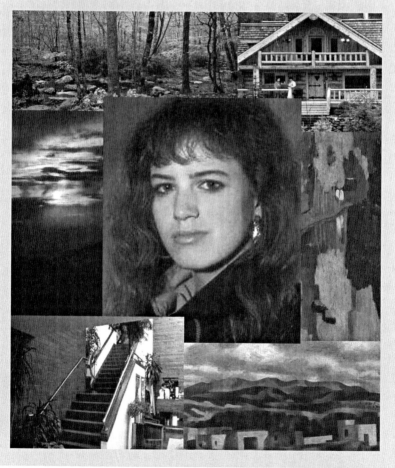

DEEP YANG

Five basic hues with golden yellow added. They are deeply saturated, blended, muted or dusty.

Cosmetics

Dark-hair *Deeps* can use more dramatic make-up, but lighter-hair *Deeps* are best in subtle, blended make-up.

Foundation: Yellow or gold-toned beige, bronze.

Lipstick/nail Colour: Orange red, peach or deep coral, mocha, brownish tones, metallic (bronze or copper). Avoid pink.

Blusher: Deep peach or apricot, coral, bronze.

Eye Shadow: Browns, warm beige, gold, muted green, bronze or copper, smoked turquoise. Add warm brown, if too bright.

Hair Colour: Red, gold, coppery brown, or auburn tones. No frosting, and no ash tones. Colour greying hair until completely gray, then avoid blue tones.

Accessories

Shoes and Handbags: Brown tones, bone (creamy), tan, bronze, copper, olive or gold.

Hosiery: Golden beige, and tones of your palette.

Glasses: Gold metal frames, tortoise shell, or hair colour, or colours that match palette.

Jewelry: *Deep* Yang coloured women should use jewelry to bring out the highlights of their skin and hair. Gold, antique gold, copper, brass or bronze, are the metals of choice. Topaz, yellow sapphire, coral, fire opal, turquoise, sardonyx, smoky quartz and tortoise shell are your best gemstones. Creamy-coloured pearls and amber-coloured jewelry are both acceptable.

Deep Yang Colouring

A *Deep's* colouring is intensely saturated with a golden hue. They have rich deep eyes and warm toned hair that is luminous. No blue eyes in this colour group.

Think of rich harvest colours and brown earth tones. Colours are mostly muted, but some are vivid. They may be mellow and rich, but always warm. In the *Deep* palette, there are no pure, primary colours. All of these colours are blends.

Colours To Wear

Reds: All reds must have yellow or orange in them. No pink, no blue-red

Pink: No pink but a rich Salmon colour

Purple: Rich eggplant purple with brown in it

Orange: Vivid or muted, pumpkin to terra cotta. Deep peach, or apricot.

Green: Yellow-greens, rich or greyed, olive, khaki, medium to deep forest green

Blue: Deep muted with green in them. Periwinkle, rich bluish purple. No clear, blue navy

Yellow: Gold tones, light to dark

Brown: Most browns, golden to chocolate. Warm beige, rust, camel, copper and bronze

Black: Warm olive or brown black, no gray

White: Off white, beige-toned

Good Basic Colours are: Beige, tan, brown, khaki, rust, coral, gold and deep forest green

A Deep Yang's Basic Colour Wardrobe

Work Wear:	Winter	Summer
Jacket	Olive Green	Oyster White
Skirt	Olive Green	Oyster White
Pants	Rust	Olive Green
Dress	Rust	Deep Lime Green
Blouse 1	Terra Cotta	Yellow Gold
Blouse 2	Green, Rust & Orange-Red	Coffee Print Green & Beige
Dressy Blouse	Warm Beige	Salmon
Sweater	Forest Green	Olive Green
Cocktail Pants	Dark Brown	Beige
Skirt Or Dress	Dark Brown	Beige

Casual Wear:	Winter	Summer
Casual Pants	Forest Green	Camel
Casual Skirt	Forest Green	Camel
Casual Top	Jade	Orange
Coat	Drk. Cocoa Brown	Oyster White
Trench Coat	Drk Warm Beige	Ivory
Evening Wrap	Drk. Cocoa Brown	Beige

Now that you have a better understanding of each Colour Harmonic group, you may have discovered that you are attracted to some of the colours in an opposite CH ruler group. The key to mixing colours is to use your power neutrals as your main colour and introduce your opposite colours in prints or accessories. Just ensure that your colour stays next to your face to look your best.

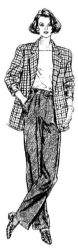

If you are attracted to colours opposite to your colour group ie: Strongs that love some of the Deep Yang colours, introduce them into your wardrobe via prints. Use your black background neutral and add brown, orange or rust red and olive in the print. Keep the scale of the print in keeping with your body size and clothing personality and you will have accomplished your goal.

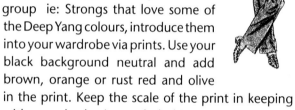

In the next section we will discover that it takes more than understanding and wearing our ruling colours. Its time to learn, accept and love our unique body shape.

We are all basically cut from four different shapes. Of course there are numerous twists and turns along with length and width differences that add spice and variety to that chosen shape.

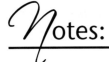

Notes:

To help you ascertain that you really understand your colouring, ask yourself these two questions:

When traveling on vacation for two weeks which two colours would I wear if they were all I could bring?

When traveling for work for a one week stretch which two colours would I wear if they were all I could bring?

STEP 3

*U*nderstand Your Body Shape

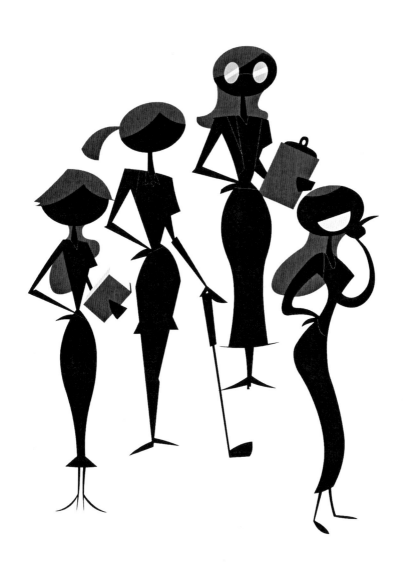

Mirror, Mirror on my plate
I see an image
that I hate

Oh what must I do
to stop the curse
of curly hair
and even worse

Small bosom & too wide hips
legs too long
and waist too thick
too thin brows, hair and lips
pendicures, manicures and waxes
to make me slick

Mirror, Mirror what do I see
is the reflected image really me?
I look good, why even nice
so pretty I had to look twice!

$\mathcal{S}$tep 3: Understand Your Body Shape

Body Shapes – What Am I?

Body type theories have been around for ages. Many are quite scientific and intricate in nature and others are more subjective. Following are a few of the well known theories and images for the different body types. If you would like to read more about them, books and website links are provided in the index area.

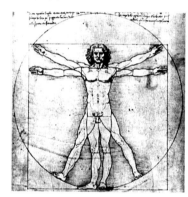

The Vitruvian Man, as drawn by Leonardo da Vinci in 1490, is based upon an earlier work by the Roman architect Vitruvius, illustrating the "ideal proportions" of the human body framed within a square and a circle. (Others placed the square exactly within the circle, but Leonardo used his extensive data to break this principle with his square no longer exactly within the circle in order to obtain more aesthetic proportions.) So the foundations for the design of modern fashions lie in creating at least the illusion of ideal proportions for the human body based upon the concept of our "collective unconscious" and its definition of ideal beauty as proposed by Carl Gustav Jung?

Balance Not Symmetry

The basic premise of this book recognizes that there are polar opposites in this world. Again, *Yin* and *Yang* will be incorporated. Some examples of this theory as seen in nature are the sun, considered Yang, and the moon is Yin. The most obvious are the human male – Yang and *female* – Yin. Within those two categories lie varying degrees of Yin and Yang. Some examples in nature are: dogs are Yang and cats are Yin. Oak trees are Yang and Willow trees Yin. Think of Yang as strong and Yin as supple.

This Is How It Works

Some people are extremely one or the other. Others are a mixture. We will be finding out where you fit on the *Ying* scale. Then we will have a starting point to find out who we really are, and why we are that way. OK, let's look at some extreme *Yin* features as seen on the human body:

YIN Physical Attributes
Petite; curvy body shape; rounded delicate bone structure.
large, rounded eyes; sloped or tapered shoulders; waist line always evident; small hands and feet; delicate skin and fine textured hair

Basic Essence
Alluring; Receptive* Charming * Artistic *Accommodating
* Diplomatic * Very Appealing Nature * Magnetic

Celebrity Examples
Elizabeth Taylor * Marilyn Monroe * Dolly Parton * Pamela Anderson* Angelina Jolie * Selma Hayek

Now, what do *Yang* Features look like?

Yang Physical Attributes
Tall, angular, broad or sharp bones; straight body lines; square shoulders – large hands and feet; blunt jawbone – prominent nose or facial features extreme texture to hair

Basic Essence
"Regally imposing" dominant * charismatic * creative * forceful * bold * commanding

Celebrity Examples
Cher * Christie Brinkly * Cybil Sheppard * Britt Eckland * Katherine Hepburn * Barbara Streisand

Some of us are taller and put weight on in different places yet, our frame or bone structure stays the same no matter how much weight we lose or gain. The sooner we accept the limitations of our unique body structure which includes; height, large or small bones, large or small hips, waist or bust area, the sooner we can move on and learn how to love the body we were born with and dress realistically to enhance who we are.

First realize that as we age, our body-shapes change due to a gradual shift in body composition. Bone structure, internal organs, body fat, and skeletal muscle tissue determine this shape. Only two of these can be modified - body fat and skeletal muscle tissue. For women, each year after the age of twenty, fat replaces half a pound of muscle weight. This means that even if you keep the same weight, a woman will have added ten pounds of body fat by age 40. This is what causes us to cringe when we see ourselves in a swimsuit.

So this is why, even when we have lost all the weight we felt we needed to lose, we still don't look like the 'Model' image we thought we would. Dieting alone will not change this natural phenomenon, but exercise and strength training can. The most important components of a fitness program are muscle strength, cardio-respiratory efficiency, flexibility, and acceptable levels of body fat. To keep that young and fit look you need to combine low impact aerobics with body sculpting exercises.

Let's Learn How To Measure Up Your Body

Understanding your body shape is the first step in figuring out how to enhance it. The following is an example of measurements taken from the model on page 86. You can fill out your own measurements on page 166 in Step 8.

Model's Height:	64"
Top of the head to Hip Bone (pivot joint):	34"
Hip Bone to the Floor:	30"

If measurements are **Equal** = You are **Evenly Proportioned**. If head to hip measurement greater = You are **Short Legged**. If hip to floor measurement greater = You are **Long Legged**.
The model above is: **Short Legged**

Waist Line Measurement:
Measure from the crease of the underarm to hipbone: (Don't raise your arms)	18"
Determine where natural waist appears and Measure from your underarm to your waist:	10"
From waist to your hip bone (pelvic hinge bone):	8"

An **Evenly-proportioned** waist falls halfway between your underarm and your hip. If underarm to waist measurement is less than waist to hipbone = You are **Short Waisted**. If measurement is greater from underarm to waist than waist to hipbone = You are **Long Waisted**.
The model above is: **Long Waisted**

Hips And Waist:
BUST Measurement:	38"
WAIST Measurement:	28"
HIP Measurement - (fullest part at pivot bone):	38"

On an average body, the hips will measure 2" more than the bust, and

9-10" more than the waist.
The model on page 86 has: **_Small Hips_**

Bust Measurement:

Fullest part of breasts and straight across your back: 38"
The chest measurement just below the breast is: 32"
Subtract this measurement from the first: 6"

If bust measurement is less than 1" larger than chest measurement = You
are *Small Busted.* If measurement is 1-3" larger than chest measurement
= Your bust size is *Average.* If measurement is larger than 3" of chest size
= You are *Large Busted.*

This is a guide to cup size: *Small* -"A" cup; *Average* - "B" or "C" cup; *Large*
- "D" cup or larger e.g.: A 34" (chest) & 36" (bust) = a 34C bra size.
The model above is: **_Large busted and needs a size 32D bra_**

Shoulder Measurement:

The circumference of the shoulder relative to the hips is:
Circumference of shoulders: 40"
Circumference of hips: 38"

Consider Equal Width of shoulders to width of hips = Average. Wider
shoulder measurement than hips = Broad Shoulders. Shoulders that are
less than hip measurement = Narrow Shoulders.
The model above has: **_Broad Shoulders_**

Now go back to the figure drawing, and transfer all the measurements
that you have received here, to the appropriate spots. You will instantly
see why you may need longer pant length or arm length in jacket or need
them hemmed up as the case may be. With this overview, you should be
able to see and understand why some styles will look more flattering on
you, than other styles. Armed with this information, you will save time
and energy when looking for new outfits, or assembling your old ones.

THE PERFECT BODY IS DIVIDED INTO FOUR EQUAL PARTS:
Nobody is Perfect....

Your body is unique. By taking accurate measurements you will know what type
of clothing will best enhance your particular structure or body shape.

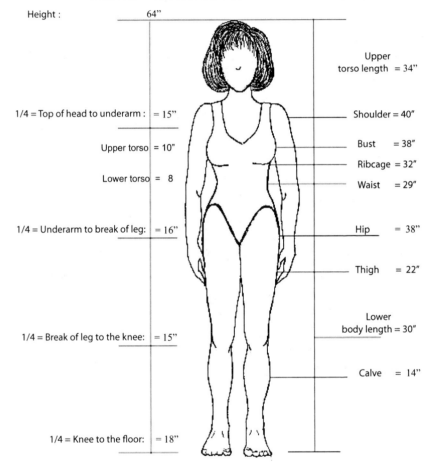

Height :   64"

1/4 = Top of head to underarm : = 15"

Upper torso = 10"

Lower torso = 8

1/4 = Underarm to break of leg: = 16"

1/4 = Break of leg to the knee: = 15"

1/4 = Knee to the floor: = 18"

Upper
torso length = 34"

Shoulder = 40"

Bust   = 38"

Ribcage = 32"

Waist   = 29"

Hip   = 38"

Thigh   = 22"

Lower
body length = 30"

Calve   = 14"

We now have a basic understanding of body type structure and know
how to properly measure our body. The next page describes the four
basic body shapes.

Straight Body Shape

*Your shoulder width may be narrower than your hips with a straight and sharper angle to them. You appear taller than you really are.

*Weight goes on your hips and thighs. You may take on a decidedly PEAR shape.

*You may have a rectangular, diamond or triangular face shape.

*You tend to be a very analytical and fastidious person that likes a sense of purpose and form over comfort.

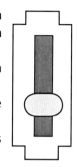

Substantial Body Shape

*Your shoulder width will be square and wider than your hip area. You tend to gain muscle easily. You become barrel-chested and square looking when you gain weight.

*You have a square, rectangular, or triangular-shaped face.

*You tend to be a very active person that likes function, efficiency and comfort over all else.

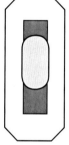

Symmetrical Body Shape

*You are average height. Your shoulders are the same size as your hips or slightly wider or narrower. You have a curved waist-line and tend to a pot belly. You can be 10 lbs. overweight before anyone notices as you put on weight equally.

*Your face shape is likely an oval, soft-edged square, or rectangular.

*You tend to be a practical person that likes structure and organization but also needs a sense of comfort. Therefore, form and function play equal parts for you.

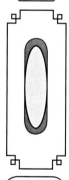

Spherical Body Shape

*You are of average height to petite. Your shoulders are round not square. You may feel overweight even when you are not. Weight goes to fleshy areas like your face, hips, or thighs but you always have a defined waistline.

*Your face shape tends towards round, oval or heart shaped.

*You tend to be a very communicative person that is very tactile. Having a free form artistic expression in all you wear or do is your mantra.

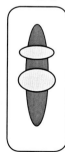

Next, learn how colours textures, size and shape of patterns used in garments have a direct effect on the type of silhouette and image you project.

Dividing Space To Create Balance

Value: the use of positive or negative space in garments to balance. For example, when space is evenly horizontally divided, this shortens, widens, and squares off the garment.

When using an uneven or unequal division of space, this creates the illusion of length. (The greater the difference between the top and bottom section of clothing, the taller the body will appear. The waist is a good stop, as it is normally less than 1/2 way on the body.)

The use of colour blocking on a garment works in an even more pronounced way, e.g., light colours and large patterns create width and attract attention. Conversely, medium to dark colours and smaller patterns, (in proper balance to body type), narrows and gives the illusion of receding or diminishing size.

*Note: Whenever a horizontal line is drawn, this will bring attention to that particular spot on the body.

Texture Use In Garments

Obvious textures like tweeds, herringbone, etc., expand space. Shiny surfaces, like satin or polished chintz, do so as well.

Soft pile fabrics such as velvet, terry cloth or corduroy also create the illusion of taking up more space because of the way light is absorbed in the folds, than is reflected at the surface.

Rough-textured, stiff or crisp fabrics suggest bulk. These fabrics are mainly be used for outer garments in more vertical-lined silhouettes, as they also hide our lumps and bumps. Pliable fabrics like knits emphasize contours, so if you do not want yours accentuated, it is best to avoid them!

Pattern Use In Garments

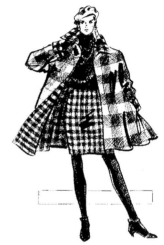

When determining a pattern use, remember - filled space appears greater than unfilled space. For example, the greater the distance between stripes, be they vertical or horizontal, the wider the whole garment will appear.

Vertical patterns or stripes are very elongating if the garment is straight cut, and a stiffer fabric is used. If a soft fabric or flowing structure is used, curves are emphasized as the vertical line now appears horizontal - cutting the elongating look that was originally intended.

If plaids, checks or prints are used, make sure that the size of the print relates and balances with your body size (Smaller prints for smaller bodies, larger prints for larger frames).

Medium sized patterns using harmonizing rather than contrasting colours are the most becoming on all body types.

Use your predetermined CH "power neutrals" in monochromatic layering to achieve a total pulled together look.

Here are some examples:
Strong Yin - black pants, charcoal top with a black and charcoal textured jacket; Subtle Yin - charcoal pants, soft white top with soft blue grey and

charcoal print jacket; Deep Yang - brown pants, tan top and a brown/ rust textured jacket; Bright Yang - beige pants, ivory top and tan, ivory and coral textured or print jacket.

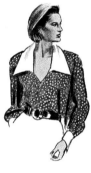

As a rule, the use of one colour in a garment or outfit is the most elongating.

The reason behind this is that the eye has no place to stop - except the face (which is where we would like it to stop)! Medium to dark colours, especially from the cool side of the spectrum, allow the garment to recede.

Light colours - pastel or vivid, especially from the warm side of the spectrum, emphasize or draw attention to the garment. This can also create the illusion of a larger space. Be careful where you use these colours.

Use light colours to expand a narrow bodice or very narrow hips. Don't use if you are trying to de-emphasize a particular figure problem! The use of contrasting colours, when done properly, can be quite effective for drawing attention to your face.

Example: lighter collars and necklines on a blouse or sweater.

The use of colours that harmonize and enhance your natural colouring can really help create the most flattering effect when combined with your figure balancing styled clothes!

The next section describes how the line of a garment visually creates a distinct image.

Clothing Lines That Create Balance

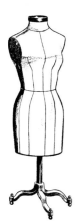

Dominant Line Of Clothing: This is the outline or silhouette of the garment. This line should compliment the natural body shape and be used to balance your body form.

Accent Lines: are lines used to attract the eye or distract the eye from looking where we don't want it to. These include top stitching, darts, accent colour bands, etc.

Vertical Lines: these lines create the illusion of length or height. A thinner look is created when properly placing vertical lines in, or on a garment.

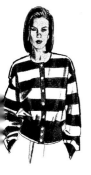

Horizontal Lines: these lines stop the eye from moving up. They create a feeling of width, and used appropriately, can make narrow shoulders appear broad, or allow narrow hips to look balanced with broad shoulders. On the reverse side, if used improperly, they can create width where we really don't want it!

Diagonal Lines: these lines suggest movement, allowing the eye to move upwards, creating a slim line on a body.

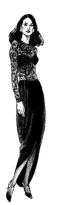

Oblique Lines: are used to create a feeling of width or narrowness, depending on how they are positioned. This is especially noticeable on garments like wrap-around tops or skirts. Also, when the tied edge is dropped at an angle on the side, this adds another slimming factor as your eye tends to stop at that point not at the horizontal line of the garment.

Notes:

Now that you have gained a better understanding of the components making up a body structure, write a paragraph that best describes your body shape uniqueness.

My body shape is.....

STEP 4

Uncover Your Clothing Personality

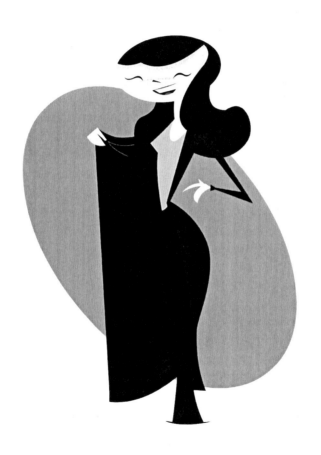

Mirror, mirror in the hall
Clothes displayed on the wall
Which item should I try
pleasing to my eye

I feel youthful
even though I'm mature
I want to feel beautiful
without turning hauteur

Clothes that defy gravity
to make me look pretty
Garments made to lift and push
while squeezing in a bountiful tush

I want to create WoWs
without lifting brows
What is my clothing style
to go the long mile

Time to take the test
to find the look that's best
A style that's mine
will save me money and time

Mirror, Mirror what do I see
A beautiful reflection
of the real me..........

$\mathcal{S}$ tep 4: Uncover Your Clothing Personality

In this step to G.U.R.U. we are going to help uncover your clothing personality style.

This area of our life can cause a great deal of unnecessary stress if we are trying to keep up to fashion trends. Most of us over 30 neither have the time, interest and/or resources to keep up to the latest look. Unless of course you are in this or another industry that requires this awareness. I'll go one step further and bet you gravitate towards certain comfort colours and styles in clothing and only purchase items that compliment those.

> This area of our life can cause a great deal of unnecessary stress if we are trying to keep up to fashion trends.

Awareness and eventual change usually comes if you have been forced by circumstance to look at how you project yourself. Maybe something wonderful has happened in your life like a new career, relationship or baby. Or, heaven forbid, a traumatic event in your life like a death of a spouse or divorce; move to a new location and/or career change. Now addressing this area of personal image is critical to ensure that you are mirroring this new "phoenix from the fire".

In the next few pages I will show you an example of a completed clothing personality quiz. The client's dominant style is uncovered in the corresponding information. The clothing personality quiz is divided into nine key sections meant to help you identify the clothing you feel most comfortable in under different circumstances. There is a blank quiz for you to personally fill out in on page 156 in Step 8.

As you continue on this journey, you will start to see a pattern develop, your personal style pattern.

Clothing Personality Style Quiz

This quiz was completed by a client identifying her **Clothing Personality Style**. She answered the questions spontaneously, and marked **One** choice in each group. At the end of this exercise, the total amounts of a's, b's, c's & d's were recorded. The largest number was her dominant clothing style and the next largest number, her secondary clothing style.

1. My favourite hairstyle is:
    ____a. Simple, sleek or asymmetrical
    ____b. Feminine style, soft curls or curves
    _√_c. Casual, with a windblown, natural look
    ____d. Controlled hair style, neat but not severe

2. The clothes I most love to wear are:
    ____a. The latest clean lined trends
    ____b. One or two piece dressy outfits
    ____c. Separates - shirts, pants, skirts
    _√_d. Tailored suits, or co-ordinated suit type looks

3. My favourite fabrics are:
    ____a. Rich, tailored, hard-finished fabrics of quality
    _√_b. Jersey, or soft-flowing fabrics with movement
    ____c. Natural fabrics of comfort; raw silk, linen, cotton
    ____d. Natural fabrics - silk, wool or rayon that keep their form

4. Dressing for a lunch date with a friend:
    ____a. Bold, eye-catching outfits that draw attention
    ____b. Soft & feminine, preferably a dress
    ____c. Jeans or casual pants, with a blouse or T-shirt
    _√_d. Tailored, suit look ensemble - monochromatic

5. Dressing for an evening out:
    ____a. Silky evening pants with a striking top in latest style
    ____b. A dress to suit the occasion
    ____c. Dressy slacks, with a dressy blouse or sweater
    _√_d. Dressy suit, tailored for the occasion

6. My favourite blouse or top is:
____a. Exotic print or coloured fabric or high style
_√_b. Femine form enhancing style with interesting detailing
____c. Jean shirt, Tee, or comfortable cotton shirt
____d. Tailored cotton, silk, or rayon blouse in a solid colour

7. The shoe I prefer to wear is:
____a. High-heeled boots or high brand quality pumps
____b. High-heeled strap sandals, or funky shoes
_√_c. Comfortable flats or low-heeled shoes or boots
____d. Leather boots (with pants), or classic closed pumps

8. The jewelry I love to wear is:
____a. Bold, sleek jewelry of value
____b. Delicate, Artsy or vintage pieces
____c. Simple, natural stone or engraved metal
_√_d. Fine quality, heritage or simple classic pieces

9. The overall image I like to project is:
____a. Polished, Planned and Sophisticated
____b. Soft and feminine with a sense of funky whimsy
_√_c. Carefree, informal, relaxed and comfortable
____d. Understated, poised and presentable for all occasions.

TOTALS:
a.__0__   b.__2__   c.__3__   d.__4__

POLISHED   ARTSY   NATURAL   CLASSIC

DOMINANT STYLE: __Classic__

SECONDARY STYLE: __Natural__

Personal Style In Clothes

Clothes are your way of letting the world see you for who you are. Whether you like it or not, people judge you by what you wear. It may not be right but, if you are honest with yourself, you will recognize that you do this as well.

Clothes tell others about your status, background and possibly what your personal lifestyle is like.

Style is more than just personal colouring or the clothes you wear.

When you understand this ahead of time, you will be able to enter a room and make a positive first impression. I am sure that everyone has heard the expression "you never get a second chance at a first impression." This is true but that doesn't mean that if you made a bad first impression that you are cursed for the rest of your life.

Don't panic. Your style will develop gradually as you begin to use all the information in this book to build your very own personal style. Style is more than just personal colouring or the clothes you wear. It is your bearing, grooming, mannerisms and the way you project your inner self!

*Please Remember:

1. Don't let your clothes say something you do not want to convey about yourself.

2. Keep it simple, but try new looks that flatter your body and personality.

3. If your clothes enhance your personality, not alter it, you have truly mastered the art of dressing.

Clothing styles have transformed over the years to reflect change. Witness the amount of external world and cultural changes that have taken place since the turn of the 20th century. Where external change happens, personal inward changes also occur.

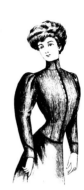

In North America during the times of World War I and II, the role of women (traditional house wife and mother), was expanded to include working outside their home in schools, hospitals, offices, and factories to keep the economy flowing while their spouses were overseas tending to world peace. This started an interest in career fashion.

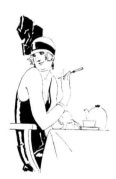

With a taste of being the bread winner at home, the revolution was on. The fashion of the twenties, thirties and forties displayed this.

In north America the fifties, sixties and seventies brought with it prosperity, peace movements and rebellion. These attitudes took a backseat in the eighties and nineties and we became more self indulgent and then cocooned ourselves.

With the 21st century still in its infancy, the evolution of expression is sure to continue. As the future unfolds, world economy, industry and education will become truly global. Our personal style will incorporate colour, fabrics and styles from all countries and ethnic backgrounds. A global rather than regional style will evolve.

This evolution of style will require a real understanding of your inner traits, clothing personality, personal colouring and body shape to allow you to not only stay individual but continue to be authentically you.

The Polished Look

If you picked *Polished* as your clothing style, and your body shape is Straight, then you will find that this description will fit you perfectly.

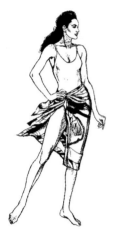

The Polished style is *Yang* in nature, strong and beautiful. You are probably on the tall side. Even if you are of average height, people will always think of you as tall. The reason for this is that your bone structure or body shape is quite narrow for your size.

Therefore, your vertical line will appear taller because of this. You tend to have long narrow and sinewy arms, legs, hands and feet. Usually, you will have sharp, square, and narrow shoulders. Your face shape will probably be either rectangular, diamond or heart-shaped, though always longer than wider. Your hair will be of extreme texture; very fine and silky (either poker straight, or with a bend) or, it could be very coarse and wavy.

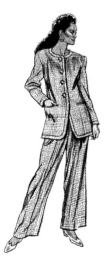

You have probably noticed that any weight you gain will first appear from the waist down with this weight stubbornly lodging itself on your hips and thighs. If you become extremely overweight, you may take on a decidedly *Pear* shape. Even when you are poker thin, you have wide hipbones but a flatter derriere. You have probably lamented over having prominent facial features. They may be a forceful jawbone, sharp cheekbones, or an outstanding nose. 'Polished' women have a tendency to feel less than beautiful, because they focus on the offending feature, when in fact; those are some of the most sought after features in photography!

Some of the most beautiful models and actresses are Straight body shapes with a Polished air about them ie:

Cher, Joan Crawford, Lauren Bacall, Lena Horne, Connie Sellecca, just to name a few. Male actors Male actors that classify as Straight, are: Pierce Brosnan, Ted Danson, Eddie Murphy.

Important "Polished" Enhancements

Shape is your most important feature. Strong, geometric shapes such as squares, triangles and rectangles are the best shapes for your clothing and accessories.

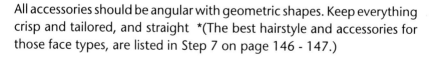

Your hairstyle, makeup and eyeglasses should be sleek and sculpted, with crisp edges. The key is to enhance your Yang features, not hide or mask them. The fabrics you are most attracted to, will have a defined shape. No flowing fabrics, use medium to heavy weight and tightly woven fabrics, with a matte, or smooth surface, to bring out the best look for you. Any colouring group is possible, high contrast or blended. When dealing with colour, think head-to-toe ensemble. Monochromatic looks add to your regal presence.

All your clothes are structured. The jackets and tops you wear should have shoulder pads in them to balance off your hip line. Not only do the pads balance your narrow shoulders, they also create a slimming illusion. Pants and skirts should be straight and tailored without horizontal pockets. Avoid using draped pants or full skirts.

All accessories should be angular with geometric shapes. Keep everything crisp and tailored, and straight *(The best hairstyle and accessories for those face types, are listed in Step 7 on page 146 - 147.)

Polished men like to wear the latest styles and trends in clothes. They like tailored, European-cut suits like Armani. They like very structured and high-class clothes. If they wear jeans, you can bet that they will be designer jeans!

The Natural

If your dominant clothing Style is **Natural**, and your body shape is Substantial, then the following information will fit you to the "T".

Your **Natural** style is also **Yang** in nature. You have a commanding presence but are commonly misjudged. You are really a jolly giant that wants everyone to feel welcome.

You are probably on the tall side. When asked, most people may think you are shorter than you are because your bone structure is broader than it is long.

When you gain weight, you will have a tendency towards becoming barrel chested. Your legs tend to be muscular. A top heavy appearance is your structure challenge. You are often considered to be quite athletic looking even if you aren't!

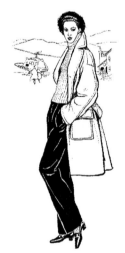

You will tend to have a square, oblong or triangular-shaped face. Therefore the best hairstyle, glasses, etc. for you are listed in the *Face Shape* section in Step 7. You are a free-spirited person that likes comfort over all else. This would include a casual wind-blown look in your hair. Little to no makeup as well as clothes that don't restrict your natural flow are the ticket.

Celebrity Examples: Christie Brinkley, Linda Evans, Cybill Sheperd, Tom Selleck, Brian Denahee, Arnold Schwarzenegger.

You will tend to gravitate towards casual separates in your clothing, items such as shirts and jackets. Pants and sweaters and loosely structured tops will probably be your mainstay clothing items. You like medium to very textured fabrics in natural fibres, especially cotton. Other appropriate fabrics are jersey, gabardine, hand-knits, corduroy, suede, and leather, as well as wool tweeds. Summer fabrics include cotton, rough linen, gauze, and raw silk. You may enjoy plaids, and checks, paisley and large casual designs, especially if they are images seen in nature.

Neutrals are the backbone colours for your wardrobe. Medium to dark colours of your palette work as well.

Your body type warrants rectangular, loose fitting, boxed-off styles that enhance your basic structure. Straight man-tailored pants will balance off your broad upper body. If you wear snug fitting pants that narrow at the ankle, you will look very top heavy. Layered looks are excellent on you, and you will look very pulled together. You should use raglan-type shoulder pads to soften your broad shoulder line. Loosely structured, simple, straight skirts look best on you. Remember, balancing your body line in your clothing style, is the key to looking your best.

Natural guys love to wear jeans and comfortable shirts. For business, a box-cut, loosely structured sports jacket with suit pants is their preferred garb. They hate anything that is overly structured. They want to wear clothes that are comfortable, not restrictive.

The Classic

If your body shape is Symmetrical and your clothing personality style is *Classic*, then what follows, will ring true to you.

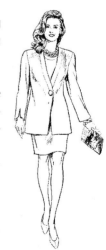

Your body shape and image style puts you in the middle of the Yin and Yang scale. You are truly balanced between the male and female aspects that all have. Some people carry more of the feminine on the outside, and masculine on the inside. Others are vice versa. Then there are those that have an equal amount of both, inside and out. This is you.

You are of average height. Most people can guess your height right on. Your most noticeable traits are that you are symmetrical. This applies to almost everything. When you gain weight, you can be 10 pounds overweight before anyone notices. Conversely, you have to lose 10 pounds before anyone notices this as well. Your face will most likely be a soft-edged square, rectangular shape, or oval. You like to have a simple, soft, sculpted hairstyle that is either straight, or has a controlled curl. Medium length hair that accentuates your face shape is what you find most flattering and comfortable.

A *Classic* is fashionable, never trendy or faddish. You like simple, tailored, structured designs in natural fabrics. Cotton, silk, wool or rayon are your preferences. You believe in quality in your wardrobe, preferring the timeless basics, to extremes in fashions, fabrics, or prints. The best way to describe your silhouette would be slight curve. Smooth, matte-finished fabrics of fine linen, wool crepe, jersey or cashmere, in light to medium weight, are best on you. Sheer or shimmery fabrics do not suit the Classic.

Most Classics prefer solids to prints, in fabrics. They will however, choose prints of medium size in stripes, geometric or floral. Evening wear brings out the beautiful fabrics like soft brocades and tapestry or silks, crepes and chiffon.

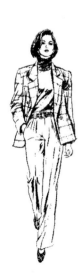

Accessories, like everything else the Classic wears, is understated and of fine quality. The key to accessorizing, is to keep it simple, not dramatic. A good quality leather handbag of medium size is best. The closed pump is the most flattering shoe style for you. If you must wear a scarf, use it at your neck only, not your hair, or waist. Pearls can be a Classic's best friend, especially if she is a Subtle Yin in colouring.

The biggest challenge that a Classic clothing personality type faces, is becoming too nondescript. Add more colour and a little drama to your wardrobe through accessories, and you will feel more powerful.

Celebrity examples: Jackie Onasis, Annette Benning, Demi Moore, and Maria Shriver. Some Male counterparts are Robert Redford, Warren Beattie, Tim Allen, and Jerry Seinfeld.

Classic men like suits, classy understated shirts and ties, as they feel best when they are in more structured clothes. Even when they dress casually, they will feel best in coordinated separates. Quality, rather than quantity, is their mantra!

The Artistic Style

If your body shape is Spherical and your clothing personality type is *Artistic*, then this is a description of you. Your image style is extreme *Yin* in nature, very feminine, soft and yielding.

Your body is curvy and possibly hourglass-shaped, which historically is the ideal feminine look. You may feel overweight even when you are not. This is because you are more fleshy than muscular. When you put on weight, it usually goes in all of the more fleshy areas such as your face, bust and hips.

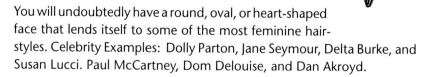

On the positive side, even when you are very overweight, you will always have a definite waistline. Conversely, even when you are at optimum weight, you will still have a fuller face, possibly but not always, a definite bust, and a fuller derriere and hips. This is a plus!

You are probably of average height, maybe even petite. Your facial features are soft and rounded. Artistics usually have beautiful eyes and facial features, and should wear colours, jewelry, and clothes that draw attention to these features. (See makeup application for the Artistic and follow your Colour Harmonics group for your best colours).

You will undoubtedly have a round, oval, or heart-shaped face that lends itself to some of the most feminine hairstyles. Celebrity Examples: Dolly Parton, Jane Seymour, Delta Burke, and Susan Lucci. Paul McCartney, Dom Delouise, and Dan Akroyd.

An Artistic loves to wear soft and flowing fabrics that make you feel graceful and feminine. Choose silk, crepe de chine, georgette, soft woolens, batiste, chiffon or gauze-like fabrics. Velvet, lace, taffeta, or satin, make beautiful evening wear.

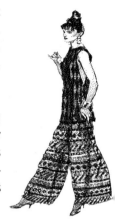

Dresses and skirts are probably your clothing mainstays. If pants are worn, they are usually soft in texture, unstructured and flowing. Blouses will be soft and flowing, possibly ruffled or embroidered. Suit fabric must be soft, and the lines gently curved.

Artistics love accessories. One must be careful not to overdo a good thing. Scarves, hair ornaments, ribbons, lace, silk flowers, beaded handbags, and strapped sandals are all part of your wardrobe. You have a tendency towards unique styles of dress. This can be on the folksy or trendy side that uses; one-of-a-kind pieces in both jewelry and clothes.

> Choose silk, crepe de chine, georgette, soft woolens, batiste, chiffon or gauze-like fabrics.

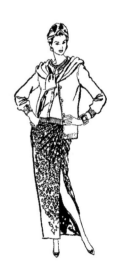

Artistic men will like the look and feel of wearing raw silk, cotton, rayon and sweaters. They will have a tendency to like wearing clothes that flow, and are comfortable, not restrictive. Artistic men can be more flamboyant than others are, and get away with it.

The Sprite

Up to this point, I have said that there are only four clothing personality styles and mentioned four body shapes. There are in fact, five.

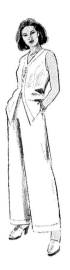

The Sprite is actually a combination of Yin and Yang living in the same body. You are petite which is Yin in stature, but you are definitely Yang in internal nature.

Every Sprite I have met has opposing inner-traits and outer-traits. They have two equal dominant inner-traits. Most often they are a Dominant Doer inner-trait with strong Mediator, Planner or Communicator inner-traits very close behind. Dynamic people in every sense of the word!

The fifth body shape can resemble any of the preceding four, with size the only real physical difference. Sprite people are the shorter, smaller, more petite forms of the other four body shapes.

You can be ruled by any Colour Harmonics group: Strong Yin or Subtle Yin; Bright Yang or Deep Yang

Your body shape could be Straight, Substantial, Symmetrical, or Spherical.

The difference in clothing style shapes is simply smaller versions of the other four types. It is very important for the Sprite to wear clothes tailored to fit their particular height, shape and form dimensions, so as not to look like a little person in big people's clothes.

> The Sprite is actually a combination of Yin and Yang living in the same body.

Your Clothing Personality Style could be Polished, Natural, Classic, or Artistic.

Notes:

In this area, describe the person you think you portray. Give this written analysis of yourself to family, close friends and associates to read. Let them honestly comment on your thoughts. I think you will be surprised with their answers.

STEP 5

Resolve Your Style Conflicts

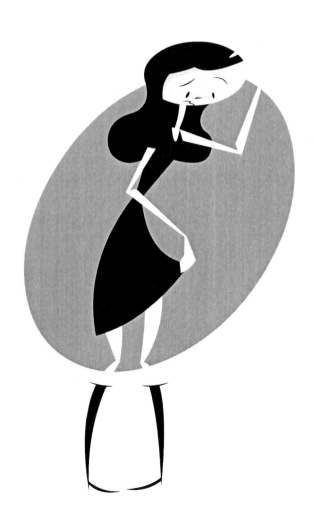

Mirror, Mirror on the wall
I ask you once
and for all...

This just can't be
this image I see
must be a mock up
of the authentic me

I am CEO of a company
That deals overseas
I need to look professional
But want to wear jeans

Where is the smile
I once knew
I must seek the child
for a clue

Mirror, Mirror now I see
the child within speaking to me,
I listen, I laugh, I love her now
A true vision of beauty
behind her once furrowed brow

$\mathcal{S}$ tep 5: Resolve Your Style Conflicts

OK, let's say you've taken the innertraits quiz and found out that you are a **Dominant Communicator**. You then filled out your clothing personality quiz and discovered that you have an **Artistic Clothing personality with Classic Admiration** (which fits with the first quiz - I will explain later) but your career role is CEO of a male dominated oil company. Do you see the conflict?

Firstly, you are Artistic and a communicator locked into a position that demands time and people management to the extreme.

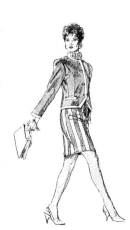

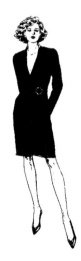

A Communicator / Artistic is who you are on the inside. You admire the Classic Clothing Personalty so take a cue from the timeless look without looking too staid for your personality.

The Corporate Image
Here is how you combine classic and artistic flare to appease you inner and outer persona as well as look impressive enough to command respect and admiration from your male coworkers.

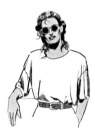

Or, what if you are a **Dominant Doer** with a **Planner** secondary and are in charge of a booking events for artists and musicians. The artists want to come in and talk. You are working on the details of promoting their careers. You are trying to get them to change their wardrobe, speech and work ethic and they want to explain to you their latest creative idea.

They think you are harsh and you think they are slackers. But, you both love your career choices.

So what can do you do to all work together? Ok, first off you need to lighten up without losing your focus. After all without your tenacity the artists won't have a place to display their works. On the other hand if you don't show that you are trying to relate to them and care about their feelings, you may lose them to another agent that is of **Communicator** or **Mediator** dominance.

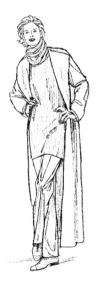

The one thing you must do is listen to their plight. The next is to dress in a manner that brings out your own creativity. You need comfortable easy to move in clothing. Create layers as it shows a sense of artistic flare that will be appreciated by your clients. Just make sure they are loose and comfortable and buy the pieces in your power neutral colours (learned about in Step 4) and viola, you have married the two styles without losing yourself in the process.

Or, maybe you are a ***Dominant Mediator*** with a ***Planner*** Secondary that was the head of the Human Resources department for a large company. You are on maternity leave as you have just started your family and now find yourself a stay at home mom.

Can you see the possible conflict here? These clothes have served you well in the past but now your biggest challenge is which day park to take your precious one for his / her morning stroll. Somehow a suit would not be appropriate here.

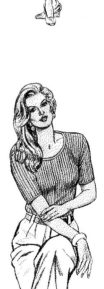

In Step 6 - Designing a full proof wardrobe will show you a great new tool called the ***Clothes Clock***. This clock will show you how to choose your daily wardrobe by charting the activities and times of day in which you will be active. An fabulous tool that makes dressing a snap.

Meanwhile, set aside the suits for now and invest in some separates that are both comfortable but stylish as well. No need to give up your Classic and timeless style just because you are working at home instead of an office.

Purchase casual pants and jeans that are slightly sculpted and figure enhancing and wear them with a top and sweater jacket to give you the corporate feel in a casual way.

Solving your wardrobe conflicts will become easier as you begin to understand who you are and the role you play during the day. If that doesn't match the "inner you," then maybe there is more to change than your wardrobe.

$\mathcal{N}$otes:

For quick reference and to solidify your knowledge thus far, jot down a sentence or two under each heading.

Your Dominant Innertrait:

Your Clothing Personality:

Your Style Challenge:

Your Style Conflict Solution:

STEP 6

$\mathcal{P}$lan a Foolproof Wardrobe

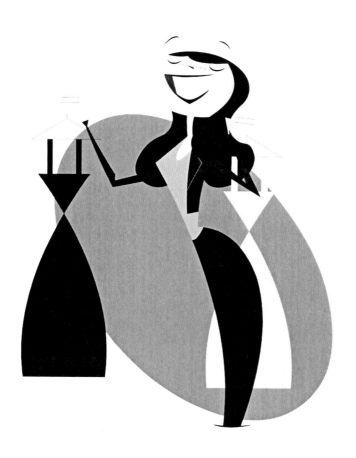

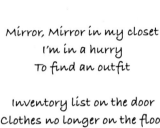

Mirror, Mirror in my closet
I'm in a hurry
To find an outfit

Inventory list on the door
Clothes no longer on the floor
Items hung and grouped by style
Shapes and colours make me smile

Jackets, pants, tops and skirts
Side by side on separate hooks
Neatly organized inside a box
Are undies, tees and tidy socks

Mirror, Mirror I feel free
Clothes Clock Complete
and totally me!

$\mathcal{S}$tep 6: Plan a Foolproof Wardrobe

In this step I will describe how to plan and build a basic working wardrobe by using a unique clock unlike the ordinary "tick, tock" that tells the time. This clock tells your wardrobe lifestyle by the hour - The **Clothes Clock**. You will also find smart & cost effective insider shopping tips to help you make good shopping decisions and avoid buying mistakes "on sale."

The normal 1am position is replaced with a 7 am start time and moves around a normal day, ending at Midnight to 6 am when the majority of us are sleeping. For those of you that aren't getting your beauty rest then, adjust your Clothes Clock to suit your own personal time schedule.

OK, now it's time to both mentally and physically clean out your closet.

Let's recap what we've learned so far:
- You now have a better understanding of what internally motivates you to react or respond.
- You know what your personal power colours are and how to use them.
- You acknowledge and applaud your unique body shape.
- You recognize your clothing personality and are now aware of any image conflicts that have arisen from this knowledge.

Because of this new awareness you are willing to change and adapt into a more authentic version of yourself.

OK, now it's time to both mentally and physically clean out your closet. This chapter will show you how to plan a working wardrobe that reflects and enhances your inner and outer body, career and lifestyle.

Journey on.........

The Pyramid Rules

Just as the Pyramid is a three-sided structure of power, majesty and balance, so can we be, if we borrow from this ideal. Remember, there is nothing new under the sun. Everything is borrowed, reworked and shared!

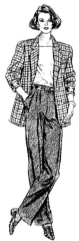

What we can learn from the pyramid is that two is good; three is balance.

For Example: If you wear a skirt or pants with a top or blouse, you have a casual look. If you wear the same outfit and add a jacket, you have created a more powerful look. How many men do you know in the corporate world that wear only a shirt and pants? They may, when they are working in their office alone. However, if their boss or a client comes in, you can bet that he has a jacket to put on, to create a more powerful and in control feeling around him!

The same is true for most women in the corporate world. It is their uniform, so to speak. The trouble arises when a women wears the wrong styled suit for her body shape. Instead of feeling in control and confident, she feels ill at ease, and can hardly wait to get home and change into a sweatshirt and yoga pants.

Granted, those clothes are comfortable, but there is no reason why your work clothes cannot be comfortable, look and fit good, as well. Gone are the days when a businesswoman could only wear a dark blue, or black suit to designate her position. She is now able to wear a large variety of timeless styles that convey her position, as well as allow her to feel like a woman, not a woman playing dress up in a man's suit.

Power Rating of Clothes

1 star* to 4 stars **** being the most powerful.

Here is a list of clothing items in order: from a formal authority position to casual clothes:

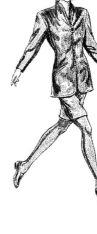

****The Matched Suit:
Jacket & skirt with a white or off-white blouse.

***The Complementary Jacket:
A dress or one colour line blouse and skirt with a long, medium, or short jacket that compliments the other pieces in style and colour.

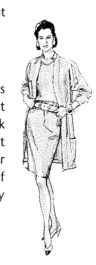

**The Complementary Patterned Jacket:
To create a less formal appearance, use a patterned jacket that has your Colour Group base and accent colours in it. Make sure that the pattern size is in keeping with your shape and size. Use your power neutrals in a monochromatic top and bottom and voila a casual but still professional look is achieved

*The Duster, Or Long Coat:
The Duster has long held a glamorous allure mainly used by Designers, Art Directors and Starlets. Think of a black tuxedo style jacket over a black straight shift dress. Or, a patterned velvet smoking jacket over satin pants. I think you get the idea. These types of jackets are not for the faint of heart as you will definitely create quite a stir.

The following items do not grade on the Power Scale:

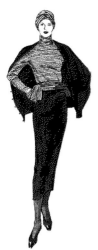

Knits

These have made a big comeback in recent years, due to the more relaxed and casual attitudes being adopted by employers and employees alike. These garment items can range from the formal and timeless Channel suits - to yoga pants combined with form fitting zippered jackets. Unfortunately, not all of our bodies are flattered in this casual style, especially for work!

Sweater Or Shrug

Over a casual pant outfit, this can dress up even a jean outfit - if selected with care. This is the most casual form of business garment accepted by employers, unless you are the boss! If this is the case, just consider who will be seeing you during the day. Will what you are wearing, add credibility and professionalism to what you do, or diminish your position?

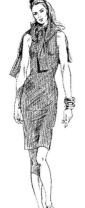

The All Important Accessories

An eye catching necklace, or scarf and earrings, with a simply cut plain dress can look just as classy as a three-piece suit. This is especially true when the colour and style enhances your body type.

The Next section displays your wardrobe lifestyle by the hour - the *Clothes Clock.*

The "CLOTHES CLOCK" tells your LIFESTYLE

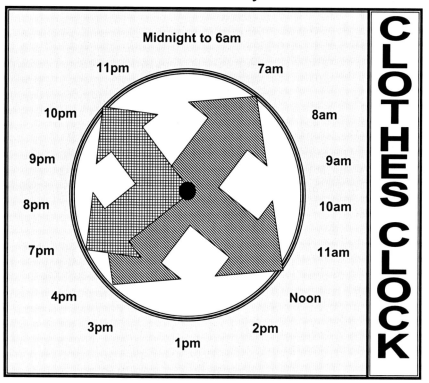

Use as many *minute & hour* arrows, filled in-between with the following GRID. This *tells* you where you spend the MOST TIME in a day and *tells* you what TYPE & STYLE of CLOTHES you should spend the MOST MONEY on when purchasing a new wardrobe.

Above example: A Mortgage Broker's "Clothes Clock"

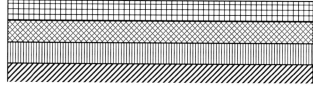

CASUAL WEAR

DRESSY CASUAL

WORK WEAR

FORMAL WEAR

The previous example of a Personal Clothes Clock displays a mortgage broker's lifestyle. She works in a high profile position where she meets perspective clients both in and out of the office.

She often (2-3x week) attends evening networking functions so her wardrobe has to move from office to evening simply. As you can see, suit type classics with shift change jackets or skirts and jewelry should make up the majority of her wardrobe.

Conversely, below is a former career woman that has chosen to take on the important role of "stay at home mom!" She would need a very different wardrobe. Right now ensuring the health and happiness of her little one is *priority one*. If however, she adopted the role of a consultant working from home, that occasionally needed to see clients, her wardrobe would have to be tweaked again to include this.

Insider Tip: Even if you are working from home it is a good idea to continue a routine of good grooming and dress to create a positive work environment.

A Stay-at-Home Mother's "CLOTHES CLOCK"

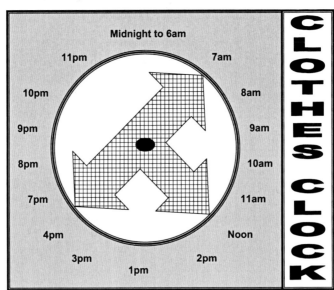

FOOLPROOF WARDROBE PLANNING

At this point, you know your **Dominant Inner-trait, Colour Ruler, and what your Body and Face Shape** is. You also know your **Clothes Clock needs.** It's time to build a real working wardrobe.

A basic wardrobe plan uses '*SEPARATES*' that '*COORDINATE*'.
Choose 2 or 3 Basic Colours from your Colour Ruler.

Here is an example list of a <u>Strong Yin's</u> power colours:

1. _____ *Black* _____
2. _____ *White* _____
3. _____ *Red* _____

2 + 2 + 5 = > 48 COORDINATING OUTFITS

2   Solid colour suits   (= two matching skirts & jackets)
+
2   Pants or skirts   (= Solid ¶ or, patterned #)
+
5   Tops   (= blouse + top + sweater + cardigan + jacket)

≥   48 Coordinated Outfits

The chart below displays the colour number and pattern symbol of clothing items in the Strong Yin's closet now. On the next page, see how these colours create a successful working wardrobe.

Two Suits	Two Pants	Two Skirts
A – 1 ¶	A – 1 ¶, #	A – 1 ¶
B - 2 #	B – 3 ¶, #	B – 3 #

Combine with any of the following: *use the key below to identify your needs*

Blouse	Top	Sweater	Cardigan	Jacket
☺ 1, 3	* 2 ¶	? 2 ¶	☺ 3 #	* 3 ¶

KEY: ☺ - Have〉   * - Need〉   ?- Want〉

Combinations of items below can create < 50 colour coordinating outfits:

CLOTHING ITEM:	COLOUR:	COMBINES WITH:
Jacket	Basic colour #1	All skirts & pants
Jacket	Basic colour #2	All skirts & pants
Skirt	Basic colour #1	All tops & jackets
Skirt	Basic colour #2	All tops & jackets
Skirt (patterned)	Coordinate #1, #2	Most jackets & blouses
Skirt or pants	Basic or accent colour #3	All jackets and blouses
Blouse (solid colour)	Basic colour #1	All skirts, pants & jackets
Blouse (solid colour)	Basic colour #2	All skirts, pants & jackets
Blouse (patterned)	Coordinate #1, #2	Most skirts, pants & jackets
Blouse or Sweater	Accent colour #3	All skirts, pants & jackets
Soft-Structured Jacket	Accent colour #3	All skirts, pants & jackets

Note: The patterned blouse and skirt could be a two-piece dress outfit.

CLOSET INVENTORY SHEET

Example: A Strong Yin's Classic Working Wardrobe

(*) Already own the item.	(!) need the item now.	(?) want the item soon

COLOURS	JACKETS	SKIRT / DRESS	PANTS	TOPS
(A) B C or D	Black White	Black White	Black White	Black White
NAVY	!	*	*	*
GREY				
YELLOW				
ORANGE				
RED	*	*	!	*
GREEN				
BLUE	!	!	!	
VIOLET				
OTHER		!Formal		
PRINTS	*!	!		*

***All clothes selected in the above section should harmonize
with the following category that was selected.**

A = Black / White	Strong Yin
B = Taupe / Off White	Subtle Yin
C = Camel / Ivory	Bright Yang
D = Brown / Beige	Deep Yang

By quick glance, you can see that this Strong Classic has her black and white basics looked after and she owns a complementary red jacket, dress and top. She also has a navy skirt and top in her style. She is now wanting to expand her wardrobe with some more colour and has chosen her CH royal blue to begin the next phase of combination outfits. She has added a formal dress to her *needs list* as she will be attending a friend's wedding in the near future. By keeping your inventory sheet up to date you can add to or cross off your list of needs simply and easily.

*Create your own closet inventory sheet using the blank copy located in Step 8 on p. 169.

The Clothes Clock Closet

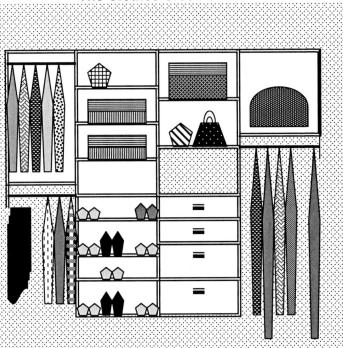

8 quick tips on designing your closet space for ease of use:
1. Layout your outfits as you would read – left to right.
2. Jackets on the top left will help select your style for the day.
3. Pants and tops on the lower left add your bottom balance.
4. Shelves of boxes filled with Tees, Scarves, belts + socks.
5. Shoes below placed 'side by side' on open shelves.
6. On upper shelves put old purses (filled with treasured items) and three basic handbags with transferable items i.e. your wallet, makeup, PDA and *Discovering your Inner Style* Journal.
7. The drawers divided + filled with underwear, bras and hose.
8. Your jewelry placed inside 'length cut' egg carton boxes (one side has individual cups for earrings and necklaces; flat side for bracelets, watches and larger items. Bonus they are stackable)
That's all there is to dressing well and feeling good.

OK, now its your turn to take the plunge. Clean out that closet! Remove, replace, and recreate your basic wardrobe to reflect your true G.U.R.U. style.

Take out everything that doesn't fit right now.
Take out all bad purchases that you've never worn.
Try on all clothes and analyze.

1. Does the item blend with my personal colours?
2. Does the style flatter my body shape?
3. Have I worn it recently (within the last year?)
4. Does the item have sentimental value?

Clothes have to look good now and always! Dated classics that are your style, but no longer current should be discarded unless they hold sentimental value.

Let's organize what is left.

a) Separate the warm and cool colours.

b) Use your CH Colour Closet Inventory Sheet* (p.169 in Step 8) as it applies to you.

c) Group all your clothing pieces together that aren't in your colours, and plan to wear these items. Don't throw them out (unless they really don't flatter you in style and fit; just add some of your right colours to them, via scarves, blouses, etc.)

d) Separate Spring/Summer clothing from Fall/Winter clothes. Place the off season clothes in a spare closet, trunk or suitcase. This will lend a bit of excitement as well, when you bring them up for the next season.

Tips On Buying Accessories

Undergarments

We need the proper foundation to build our image on. These include bras, panties, teddies, slips, stockings and shoulder pads. These items can make or break an outfit! Always bear in mind your body shape when purchasing one-piece undergarments. Are you long or short waisted? Nothing feels more uncomfortable then ill-fitting teddies or bodysuits! This also includes panties that ride up if they are the wrong size or shape for your hips and waist. Look into alternatives like G-string or V shaped boy short panties that stay put and do not ride up. Do not knock it until you try them. They are truly amazing – if the right size!

Bras

Make sure you are buying the proper size and colour of bra. The rule is to measure the circumference of your rib cage directly below your bosom. This is the BRA size. Next measure the circumference of your bust line. This becomes your CUP size – A, B, C, D, DD etc. Use your measurement guide on page 165 and 166 to ensure a snug, but comfortable fit. Because every manufacturer is different, always try them on for personal fit. Do not buy the bra just because the label lists the right size.

Stockings

Should be the same tone or lighter, never darker than your shoes or skirt or attention will be drawn to your feet.

Shoulder Pads

If used to balance the bodyline, should be as follows for each Body Shape:

Straight: Medium to larger foam, with edge cut at shoulder.

Substantial: Do not need them because you already have larger, square shoulders, but if needed, go with the Raglan style.

Symmetrical: Medium sized, soft, square-shaped pads that end at shoulder line are best.

Spherical: Small to medium-sized, rounded foam pads only. Shoulder pads are a great body-balancing tool, as well as a visual weight reducer.

Scarves & Belts

These accessories can be not only functional, but also very decorative. For effective accessorizing, keep in mind, size (scale to body), and colour (neutral or accent), or else you could create a body chopping distraction.

Shoes & Boots

These items should display quality, or they can wreck an otherwise great outfit. Quality is only one ingredient, as is the appropriate style for the outfit. For example, closed-toe pumps are always best for work. High-heeled strap sandals are party wear. Boots can also add or detract from an outfit. Use your dark, neutral colours in high-cut, high-heeled boots under long skirts, and low-cut, low to medium heeled boots with pants.

Jewelry And Hair Ornaments

Your personality can really come through in these items. For example, Polished clothing personality types can wear striking, one-of-a-kind pieces. Naturals like simple chunky chains, or uniquely cut stones on a pendant. Artistic types can wear floral and/or artsy creations and Classic types like timeless, simple pieces that speak quality.

If your body shape and your personality type are different, then accessories can show those differences, without upsetting your bodyline. For example, if your are an Artistically bent Classic, you can wear one very elaborate Victorian pin or pendant, with earrings to match. Alternatively, a Natural that has a touch of the Exotic, can wear her free style clothes with a dramatic stone necklace and earrings, or drape an exotically printed scarf over her shoulder.

Insider Tip: by Licenced Nail Technician Helen Sergiannidis
Beautifying yourself, especially having your nails done, is a simple way of feeling *"done."* Gel nails are a very low maintenance way to achieve that. Plan for 1 1/2 hours to have them put on. Fills are every four weeks (1 1/2 hours). Are you wondering what the difference is between gel and acrylic nails? Gels are non-porous and non-toxic. That's enough to convince me to choose gel over arcrylic nails!

As you may have gathered by now, I am a very practical person. In *my* "perfect world" I would like everything to be organized and easily accessible without a lot of fuss.

Here is a list of items I have in my special "just-in-case" carry all.

Personal Care Kit:

Nail clippers

Nail file

Polish remover

8 hr lipstick

Foundation

Lip-liner

Travel tooth brush

Visine

Glasses Cleaner

Sunscreen

Panti-hose – neutral

Umbrella

Plastic bags

Napkins

Clear packing tape

Change purse

Pocket mirror with magnifier

Tweezers

Clear nail polish

Dental picks

Lip gloss

Concealer

Eye, brow and white pencil

Breathe mints

Contact lens rinse

Sunglasses

Hat

Extra pair of shoes

Net carry all bag

Blanket

Feminine products

Garment brush

Note pad and pen

Add your own items:

_____

_____

_____

_____

_____

Insider Tips

When Shopping for clothes...............
1. Carry Your Image to Interior Personal Style Journal; the Colour Harmonics tool and inventory list with you at all times.

2. Don't buy impulsively!

3. Have a shopping strategy and buy at season's end.

4. Spend the most money on the clothes you'll wear the most (see your filled in Clothes Clock on p. 167)

5. Dress well when shopping: The store clerks will give you much better attention.

6. Wear or bring the foot wear and leggings you would normally wear with the outfit you are looking for to see the whole picture.

7. Use The Following As A Shopping Guideline:
> Find your size first.
> Next find your colour.
> Is it your personality?
> Does the style flatter your body shape?
> How does the fabric feel & what does it contain?
> Try the item on and check the fit. That's all there is to it.

8. Finally, find a friend that has done these exercises with you and understands the principles behind personal colouring; body type shape and the personality that will be wearing the item in the appropriate situation and your shopping experience will become an adventure, something to look forward to instead of dreaded!

Notes:

In a short paragraph, describe the clothing items you will need for the next 2 years. Make sure that you keep your colour, shape, style, Clothes Clock and inventory list at the forefront of your mind.

STEP 7

$\mathcal{R}$eveal Your Natural Beauty

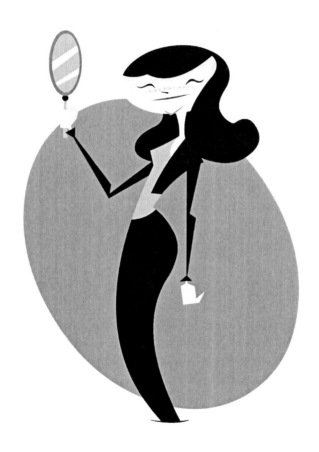

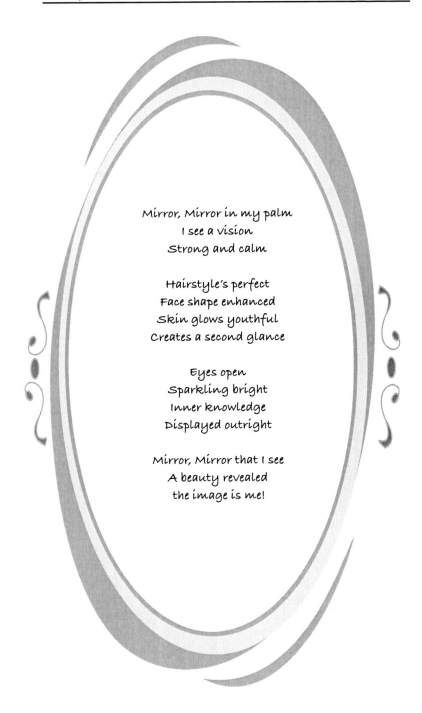

Mirror, Mirror in my palm
I see a vision
Strong and calm

Hairstyle's perfect
Face shape enhanced
Skin glows youthful
Creates a second glance

Eyes open
Sparkling bright
Inner knowledge
Displayed outright

Mirror, Mirror that I see
A beauty revealed
the image is me!

$\mathcal{S}$ tep 7: Reveal Your Natural Beauty

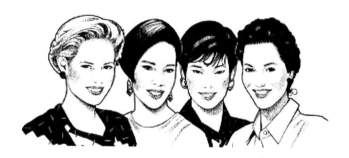

Your Face Shape

This step is about revealing your inner beauty by enhancing an authentic image for you to present to the world.

You need to recognize which face shape you have in order to augment it with the appropriate makeup and hairstyle. You could be the artist's ideal image of beauty, the Oval. Alternatively, you may have a round, square, rectangular, triangular, diamond or heart-shaped face. The "face shape measurement guide" will help you decide.

I have illustrated four different makeup styles as they relate to your inner-traits, body shape, and clothing personality style. This is an area where you can combine styles if you find you have a conflict. For instance, if you are a Classic that has a square shaped face but love the Artistic style, you can create the look of softness with a gentle wave around your face, focus on your eyes and give your lips a softer look and voila you have created an Artistically Bent Classic style!

Have fun! Remember this is play time.

BALANCED BEAUTY - THE OVAL FACE

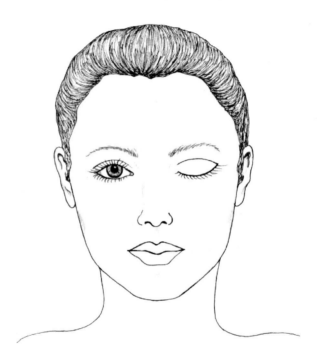

Face Shapes:

Above is an example of the historically accepted signature face shape of beauty - the Oval. There are several reasons for this:

1. Oval shapes display balance - strength with softness.

2. The balanced look is created by subtle roundness in the forehead and cheek area that tapers down to a lightly defined chin.

3. The Oval is the easiest shape to enhance with different hairstyles, makeup and accessories.

4. The Oval look is often strived for by the other face shapes. This can be achieved through specific hair styles, makeup and eyeglasses that help create the illusion of the Oval shape. The next few pages discuss flattering makeup techniques for each body shape and corresponding clothing personality style.

As can be expected by now, there are also four basic make-up techniques that correspond to the:

Four - Colour Harmonic Groups + Four Body Shapes = Four Make-up Styles & Techniques

Polished	=	Straight
Natural	=	Substantial
Classic	=	Symmetrical
Artistic	=	Spherical

Do you want to look *simple and yet striking* for the day or night on the town?
Then choose:
The Polished Face - Especially For The Straight Body Shape

Do you want to look *fresh-scrubbed, healthy, and tanned?* A look that says, "I'm a Free Spirit"?
Then choose:
The Natural Face - Especially For The Substantial Body Shape

Do you want to look elegant and refined, trustworthy and timeless?
Then choose:
The Classic Face - Especially For The Symmetrical Body Shape

Do you want to look *feminine, artistic, and soft?*
Then choose:
The Artistic Face - Especially For The Spherical Body Shape

The Polished Look: (Straight)

*FACE: Use a liquid concealer to match skin, foundation; can be light to very light. Translucent powders to create a flawless look. Highlighter under the brow and over your cheeks is effective for evening.

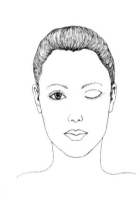

*LIPS:
- Use lip liner
- Create lips for mood
- Vibrant palette colours

*CHEEKS:
- Use little cheek colour

*EYES:
- Anything goes
- Use of vertical shadows
- Eyeliners and coloured mascara

*EYEBROWS:
- Sculpted perfectly
- Arched, not rounded
- Use your dark, *Ying* coloured eyebrow pencil

*NOTE:

The *Polished* make-up application for the *Straight* body type is as follows: Heavier application of your bright or dramatic colours for those evenings out, or use medium application and colours for any business activities. Then use a softer application of your *Colour Harmonic* - palette colours for day, at home, or play.

Natural: (Substantial)

*FACE: In order to achieve the *Natural* look, you must create a freshly scrubbed, healthy complexion. If you tan, all the better, the sun kissed look is perfect. Use a foundation a touch darker than your complexion.

*LIPS:
- Use neutral lip liner mixed with gloss to create a pouty, sexy look.

*CHEEKS:
- Use little cheek colour, blend with sponge, touch face across high points. Use a shiny powder (like a bronzer), on top of the colour.

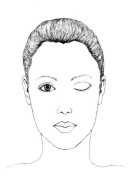

*EYES:
- Attention grabbing
- Use dusky shadows
- Soft eyeliners and lots of dark natural mascara

*EYEBROWS:
- Wild and untamed
- Straight lined, no arch
- Use your dark, *Ying* coloured eyebrow pencil

*NOTE:

The *Natural* application of make-up for the *Substantial* body type can be used in several ways: Heavier application of your dark neutrals for evenings out; medium colours and application for home and business, or use the soft peach or pink shades (depending on your *Colouring Harmonic Group)*, for that romantic evening planned.

Classic: (Symmetrical)

*FACE: To create the *Classic* look, you need to use light foundation, paler than skin. Use ivories or beige foundation well blended, for that perfect porcelain look. Use sheer powder to make a "Matte" appearance.

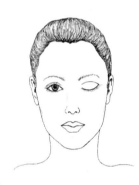

*LIPS:
- Use a dark, neutral lip liner sculpted perfectly. Matte Red is the classic colour.

*CHEEKS:
- Sculptured cheek colour
 - Use a matte powder

*EYES:
- Keep eye shadow in the crease of the eye
- Soft smudged eyeliners and dark, natural mascara

*EYEBROWS:
- Symmetrical
- Perfectly shaped
- Use your dark, *Colour Harmonic* coloured eyebrow pencil

*NOTE:

The *Classic* application of make-up for the *Symmetrical* body type can be used in a variety of ways. Use a dark neutral, or the darker colours of your palette applied in a heavier manner for evenings out; medium colours and application for home and business, or use the quieter shades of your palette softly applied (but always sculpted), for those romantic evenings.

Artistic: (Spherical)

*FACE: To create the perfect *Artistic* face you have to begin by thinking heavenly. Use tinted foundations in lavender (under base). Also use a pale pink or peachy (depending on your colouring) foundation with a sponge to blend to give that perfect porcelain doll Cherub look. Dust lightly with an opal like powder.

*LIPS:
- Think rosebud look
- Soft, rounded and dewy

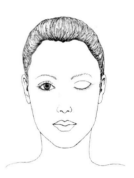

*CHEEKS:
- Think "Apple Cheeks"
- No angles, soft, rounded edges only

*EYES:
- Soft and muted colours
- Soft smudged eyeliners, mascara
- Keep shapes rounded, not harsh

*EYEBROWS:
- Use your dark, **Color Harmonic** coloured eyebrow pencil, smudged soft and rounded.

*NOTE:

The *Artistic* application of make-up for the *Spherical* body type can be used in numerous ways. Heavier application of the deeper shades will look great for evenings out; medium colours and application for business and pleasure, reserving the sexiest look softly applied for those romantic evenings with your loved one.

A More Indepth Look At Our Skin

Your skin protects the underlying tissues from radiation and any mechanical injuries. It protects against any bacteria, or other organism invasion. The sense organ maintains the body's temperature to within a few degrees of the average 98.6 degrees Fahrenheit. The skin also stores body fat, and eliminates water and salt.

The skin is composed of three layers:
> - the outer epidermis
> - the middle dermis (regulates the flow of heat)
> - the inner subcutaneous (fatty - insulator) layer

We shed millions of dead cells every day by either bathing or what rubs off on our clothing. The skin also rebuilds itself every 27 days. The process is called keratinization. The cells in the epidermis also determine the colour of a person's skin. These cells, called melanocytes, produce the pigment melanin.

What Can We Do To Ensure Healthy Skin? Firstly, let me state, that I am not promoting any particular skin care company. Each company has their own way of determining skin types. And this information allows them to know which product is best for that skin type.
The skin types are typically described as:

Normal - Clear, smooth skin neither excessively oily nor dry, and has good resiliency.

Dry - Skin is usually thinner looking, that becomes easily dehydrated, therefore more prone to wrinkles.

Oily - Skin is thicker, resilient, that has overactive sebaceous glands. These enlarge the size of the skin's pores, allowing more impurities to enter, thus causing breakouts.

Combination - This is when the majority of your skin is smooth and normal, but in the T-Zone (forehead, nose, chin) your sebaceous glands are overactive, causing shine and skin eruptions.

Skin Care - No matter which line of products you use, these steps apply. When you find the right skincare system, use all that specific company's skin care products as they work together. This is not just a marketing ploy! Use the skin questionnaire from the cosmetic company of your choice to find out what type of skin you have - normal, dry, oily or combination. The usual five-step skin care process is:

1. Cleansing   2. Toning   3. Moisturizing
4. Protecting   5. Exfoliating from 1 - 3x week.

Now, let's work on the foundation under the skin to create a clean face pallette to work on.

Background Make-up

1. Determine whether you have warm or cool-based colouring.

2. Use yellow or blue-toned colour stick to tone down imperfections.

3. Use a dot of colour on your jaw line of the foundation colour you wish to wear. If it is noticeable, *Do Not Wear It*! This will make you look like you are wearing a mask. *Do Not* wear foundation on your neck! It will wear off on your clothing, adding to your dry cleaning bill, not your beauty!

4. Once you have chosen the right colour and proper type of foundation (either for normal, oily, or combination skin), use a clean, wet sea sponge for application. Bring foundation from the forehead down, going with the hair follicles on your face, sealing in precious moisture. In addition, you will not fill up your freshly cleaned pores with colour! Finally, use your fingertips to smooth out the colour as needed.

5. Please, remember to remove all make-up before bed. Your skin needs to breathe and have time to rejuvenate itself no matter how light your make-up application is.

6. Drink up to eight glasses of pure water per day. This is your body's best friend. No matter where you live - it moves impurities out of your system and keeps your skin hydrated to look its best! If you're not a natural water drinker, fool yourself by placing up to a tablespoon of lemon or lime juice in a glass of water. Silly maybe, but it works!

How We Enhance Our Natural Beauty

Feature Make-up

1. Use make-up pencil liners to help delineate space.

2. If you wear contacts, put them on before applying any make-up - it helps to see what you are doing!

3. Apply your proper foundation colour and apply in a downward motion over your entire face.

4. Start working with your lips. This will set the tone for the rest of your make-up application (high contrast, or blended).

5. Next do the cheeks. Never crowd the nose with colour, use the center of your eye as the guideline as what not to go beyond. Always, apply cheek colour above the cheekbone never below. Use contour colour there.

6. The eyes have it next! Depending on your colour selection for your lips and cheeks (which should be very close in tone and colour), choose your eye make-up to draw people's attention to your eyes. Do them subtly or very dramatically, depending on the effect you have started with your lip and cheek colour application. * See make-up application as it applies to each body shape. Remember your eyes are the windows to your soul!

7. Your eyebrows supply the frame to your windows. Make sure they are in good shape - not too bushy, nor too sparse. You can make the necessary repairs with colour, as need be. Just ensure that you use short, delicate strokes to mimic hair.

8. Do not forget your hands. Unbelievably, the first place we women show the effect of aging, is in our hands and necks! Spoil yourselves with an occasional manicure and pedicure. It is worth it!

9. The final step to look pulled together and feeling great, is **Fragrance**. Fragrance comes in many strengths and undertones like floral, spicy, very potent to only a delicate hint of scent. Whichever is your fancy, make sure it is you. It is an important part of your overall image. Remember, expense has nothing to do with whether it enlivens or overtakes you!

Insider Tips: by Kimberly A. Pettifer

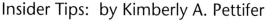

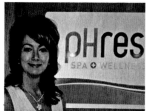

Certified licenced Estetician
Co-owner of pHresh Spa
Downtown, Vancouver, BC
604-662-4462
www.phreshspa.com

How to look pHresh when you don't feel it:

Exfoliate! Exfoliating aids in removing dead skin cells that creates both short and long-term differences in the appearance of your skin. Any lines, shadows, ageing, pigmentation differences, sun damage, colour of skin, overall youthfulness and appearance will be helped by exfoliating every two or three days. This helps your face creams work better and penetrate into the skin because the dead spongy surface layer is gone! You will also use less cream, your make-up will glide onto your skin better and last longer, thereby creating a more youthful appearance.

Another easy fix to looking tired is using highlighters or the inexpensive soft white pencil (you can get it at any drug store - look for 'West Germany'). Highlighters will help move a dark or shadowed area forward and vice versa. Dark shades will help decrease or move protruding areas backwards. Dark lines in the skin are shadows so highlight these areas. First use your highlighter under the brow line - smudged in to open the eyes. Next highlight fine lines and wrinkles with white pencil smudged in. Now apply your colour correct foundation and brush loose powder over your face to "set" the look.

Do you have dark circles under your eyes? Check your vitamins; exfoliate; or possibly look into changing your diet.

Meanwhile: Apply a light application of your skin colour foundation; place concealer where needed (the purpled areas on the skin); blot make-up with a sponge; highlight remaining areas still showing darkness; add a bit more foundation to blend and finally set with powder.

Your Face Shape Determines: Your hair style; eyeglass shape; earrings and jewelry as well as your make-up application.

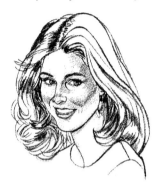

Heart-Shaped Face

You have wonderful cheekbones that can be emphasized with angular hair styles. You may wish to take width off the forehead with fullness or bangs.

Recommended Hairstyle: Minimize the width across the forehead with soft curls or bangs, and add fullness at the jawbone. Avoid styles that are shorter than the jawbone.

Choice Eyeglasses: A style that is either full, rounded or oval that extends past the cheekbones.

Right Earrings: Use styles that are rounded or irregular shaped like tear drops, to add width to the jawbone.

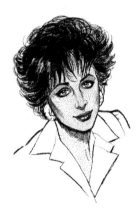

Oval Face Shape

You have the easiest face to accentuate. It is usually wider at the forehead than at the chin, with a graceful taper from cheeks to jawbone.

Recommended Hairstyle: Shoulder length or shorter styles angled at the jawbone will accentuate the curve of the cheekbones. Also, use styles that add width to the face.

Choice Eyeglasses: Any style, as long as they are wider that the widest part of the face.

Right Earrings: Use curved and angled styles, nothing too long and dangling.

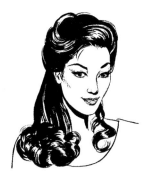

Diamond-Shaped Face

You have prominent cheekbones that need balance by styling your hair, using fullness around your temples, and in the chin area.

Recommended Hair Style: Maximizes width around the temple and use bangs or flips. The best length is chin, to middle shoulder length.

Choice Eyeglasses: Use narrow, vertical oval styling that brings attention to the center of your face.

Right Earrings: A rounded or irregular shape, like tear drops.

Round Face Shape

The round face is almost as wide as it is long. The cheekbones are not well defined.

Recommended Hairstyle: Long, layered or short styles add height to the face, but not extra width.

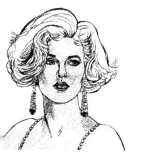

Choice Eyeglasses: Square and angular shapes that do not extend past the cheekbones, are the most flattering.

Right Earrings: Rectangular, long narrow shapes

Square Face Shape

The square face has the same height and width forehead, cheekbones and jawbone.

Recommended Hairstyle: Styles that lengthens the face and adds fullness on top. Avoid adding width at the jawbone. Emphasize angles by wearing asymmetrical and geometric cuts.

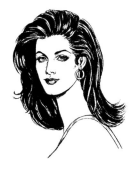

Choice Eyeglasses: Use round or oval frames

Right Earrings: Curved, longer shapes

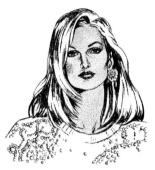

Rectangular-Shaped Face

This face shape is longer than it is wide, with about the same width across the forehead, cheekbones and jawbone.

Recommended Hairstyle: Use a style with soft bangs, to shorten the face and add width to the cheekbones. Avoid styles that add height to the top of the head.

Choice Eyeglasses: Round or oval shapes, with frames that extend past the cheekbones will diminish the width of the jawbone.

Right Earrings: Wide, round, square or fan shaped earrings help create width around the cheekbone.

On the next page is a measuring guide to assist you in determining your face shape. The measurements shown describe a rectangular face. A blank face is given for your use in the personal style appendix on page 159.

Discover your Face Shape

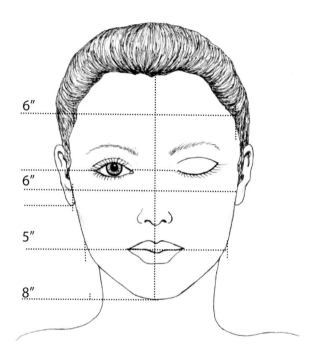

To find out the shape of your face measure it with a soft cloth tape measure. Take the following facial measurements. If you are unsure, ask a good friend or significant other to help you do the measurements.

1. Face Width __8"__ Measure your face across the top of your cheekbones. The measurement should extend from the edge of one cheekbone to the exact point on the other cheekbone.
2. Jaw Width __5"__ Measure your jaw line extending from the widest point on one side of your jaw to the widest point on the other side.
3. Forehead Width ___6"___ Measure across your forehead at the widest point. Usually the widest point will be about halfway between your eyebrows and your hairline.
4. Face Length _____8"_____ Measure from the tip of your face line to the bottom of your chin.

Insider Tips: *You and Your Hair Style by Mary Campeotto*

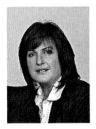

Licenced Certified Hair Stylist
Owner / Operator of Boccolli Hair
1340 Nanimo St. Vancouver, BC
604 253-3616

Frequently Asked Questions:

Q. How should decide which hair length and style you should wear?
A. A simple style that you will realistically be able to maintain after leaving the salon. Your hair style should suit you as a person and your lifestyle.

Q. I was looking through the glamor magazines and there are so many styles. How do I choose the right one?
A. Stop picking up magazines and trying to mirror the models! Ask yourself which age bracket are you in 30's to 40's; 40's to 50's; 50's to 60's ? What do you do for a living? What image you want to portray? And finally, are you being authentic for your age and experience level?

Q. How do I find a good hairstylist for myself?
A. Recommendation is always the best way. Sit in a mall and people watch. When you see someone that has a style that looks pulled together, yet natural, ask where she gets her hair done.

Q. How do I ensure a hair colour that will look good on me?
A. The short answer, depends on your personality type and trend tolerance. Have hair colour that emulates your career and experience level. When in doubt make it natural looking and harmonize with your skin tone (muted for dark skin and brighter for light coloured skin).

*Note: Be aware of how much time you will realistically need to spend on maintaining your hair colour. You don't want roots to show, especially if you are trying to cover gray. A large contrast with your natural hair colour may mean a trip to the salon every three weeks.

STEP 8

$\mathcal{E}$xpress Your True G.U.R.U. Style

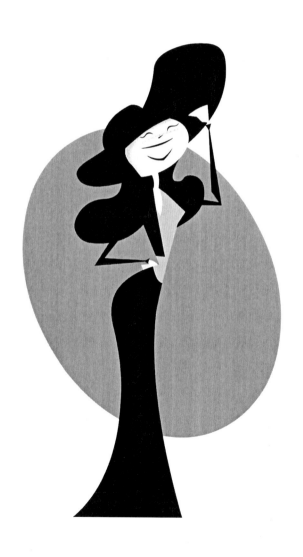

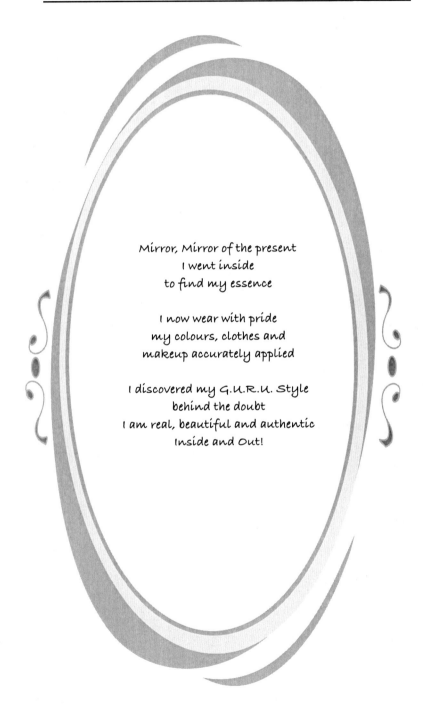

Mirror, Mirror of the present
I went inside
to find my essence

I now wear with pride
my colours, clothes and
makeup accurately applied

I discovered my G.U.R.U. Style
behind the doubt
I am real, beautiful and authentic
Inside and Out!

$\mathcal{S}$ tep 8: Express Your True G.U.R.U. Style

We have reached the final step - Step 8 to discovering your inner style. You are now becoming your own style G.U.R.U. I hope the information I've brought together in this book, that has helped me, will do the same for you! It has been a pleasure sharing it with you.

This chapter is all about you. there are blank questinaires and forma to fill out with your own information to make this a personal style journal. It may be *The End Of This Book*, but it is just the *Beginning* of the *Real You*. Take this material and use it as "the *8 Basic Stepping Stones To Reach Your True G.U.R.U. Style."*

Following is a quick reference guide to show how these subjects all relate together. Remember, this is only a guide, even though it is fairly accurate! As with anything, there are always exceptions to the rule.

Using the premise that you can be any Harmonic Colouring, now ask - if I have this category as my Dominant *Innertrait* and I am this *Body Shape* it follows that I would probably like this *Image* to *Interior Design Style.*

Innertrait	Body Shape	Image To Interior Style
Planner	Straight	Straight/Planned
Doer	Substantial	Substantial / Casual
Mediator	Symmetrical	Symmetrical / Classic
Communicator	Spherical	Spherical / Freeform
Diamond	All	Synchronistic

Describe your Inner self:

1. Which of the following personality types would you more likely emulate?

____ a. I like to work by myself. My pace is slow and methodical. I love to handle details. Some think that I border on being a perfectionist.

____ b. I don't like pushy, aggressive, types. I enjoy warm, close relationships, and I am a good team player.

____ c. I don't like to waste time. I enjoy challenges, taking control and solving problems.

____ d. I love to be the centre of attention. I like to be involved with people. I don't like to work alone, and detail work bores me to tears. I love to work with ideas and people rather than facts and figures.

2. Which of the following places would you prefer to vacation at many times?
____ a. Alone or with a close friend travelling to historic places?
____ b. In the wild mountains – Skiing, hiking or exploring? Or
____ c. In a fast paced city at all the latest restaurants, Clubs and shopping?
____ d. With your partner or family in a private cabin?

TOTALS:
a._____   b._____   c._____   d._____

PLANNER   MEDIATOR   DOER   COMMUNICATOR

Dominant Style: _____

Secondary Style:_____

The Diamond Character Locator

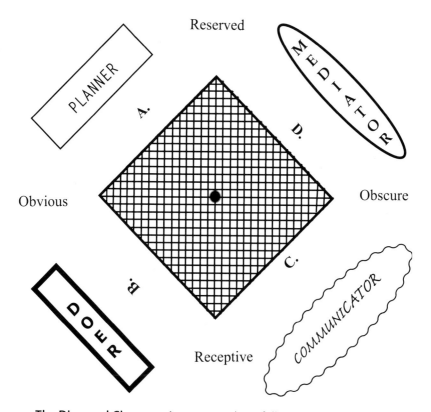

The Diamond Character Locator works as follows:

The center circle starts with a value of zero - **0**. The next line moving from the circle equals **1** - which reprepresents the *least like* **inner-trait** and **16** being the *most like* **inner-trait**. Filled-in lines create the size of *diamond* you are and also illustrates your *clarity or, response* type.

A is a **Planner**; **B** is a **Doer**; **C** is a **Communicator** and **D** is a **Mediator** personality type.

Complete your own answers from the quiz on pages 28 - 30. Insert your numbers: A = ___; B = ___; C = ___ ; and D = ____.

Your **Dominant Inner-trait** is _____and you are a _____ personality type that is both _____ and _____ about it.

Your **Secondary Inner-trait** is: _____.

Your Clothing Personality Style Quiz:

This quiz will help you identify your own *Clothing Personality Style*. Answer these questions spontaneously. Mark only **One** choice in each group. At the end of this exercise, total the amounts of as, b's, c's & d's that you marked. The largest number will be your dominant clothing style and the next largest number, your secondary clothing style.

1. My favourite hairstyle is:
____a. Simple, sleek or asymmetrical
____b. Feminine style, soft curls or curves
____c. Casual, with a windblown, natural look
____d. Controlled hair style, neat but not severe

2. The clothes I most love to wear are:
____a. The latest clean lined trends
____b. One or two piece dressy outfits
____c. Separates - shirts, pants, skirts
____d. Tailored suits, or co-ordinated suit type looks

3. My favourite fabrics are:
____a. Rich, tailored, hard-finished fabrics of quality
____b. Jersey, or soft-flowing fabrics with movement
____c. Natural fabrics of comfort; raw silk, linen, cotton
____d. Natural fabrics - silk, wool or rayon that keep their form

4. Dressing for a lunch date with a friend:
____a. Bold, eye-catching outfits that draw attention
____b. Soft & feminine, preferably a dress
____c. Jeans or casual pants, with a blouse or T-shirt
____d. Tailored, suit look ensemble - monochromatic

5. Dressing for an evening out:
____a. Silky evening pants with a striking top in latest style
____b. A dress to suit the occasion
____c. Dressy slacks, with a dressy blouse or sweater
____d. Dressy suit, tailored for the occasion

6. My favourite blouse or top is:

____a. Exotic print or coloured fabric or high style

____b. Feminine form enhancing style with interesting detailing

____c. Jean shirt, Tee, or comfortable cotton shirt

____d. Tailored cotton, silk, or rayon blouse in a solid colour

7. The shoe I lprefer to wear is:

____a. High-heeled boots or high brand quality pumps

____b. High-heeled strap sandals, or funky shoes

____c. Comfortable flats or low-heeled shoes or boots

____d. Leather boots (with pants), or classic closed pumps

8. The jewelry I love to wear is:

____a. Bold, sleek jewelry of value

____b. Delicate, Artsy or vintage pieces

____c. Simple, natural stone or engraved metal

____d. Fine quality, heritage or simple classic pieces

9. The overall image I like to project is:

____a. Polished, Planned and Sophisticated

____b. Soft and feminine with a sense of funky whimsy

____c. Carefree, informal, relaxed and comfortable

____d. Understated, poised and presentable for all occasions.

TOTALS:

a._____   b._____   c._____   d._____

POLISHED   ARTSY   NATURAL   CLASSIC

Dominant Style: _____

Secondary Style:_____

Discover your Face Shape

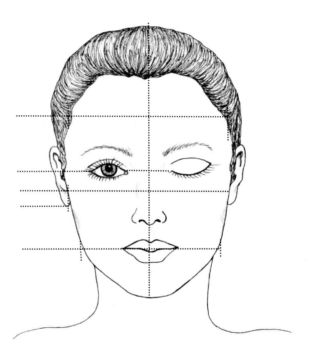

To find out the shape of your face measure it with a soft cloth tape measure. Take the following facial measurements. If you are unsure, ask a good friend or significant other to help you do the measurements.

1. Face Width _____ Measure your face across the top of your cheekbones. The measurement should extend from the edge of one cheekbone to the exact point on the other cheekbone.
2. Jaw Width _____ Measure your jaw line extending from the widest point on one side of your jaw to the widest point on the other side.
3. Forehead Width _____ Measure across your forehead at the widest point. Usually the widest point will be about halfway between your eyebrows and your hairline.
4. Face Length _____ Measure from the tip of your face line to the bottom of your chin.

Your Make-up Style Looks Like:

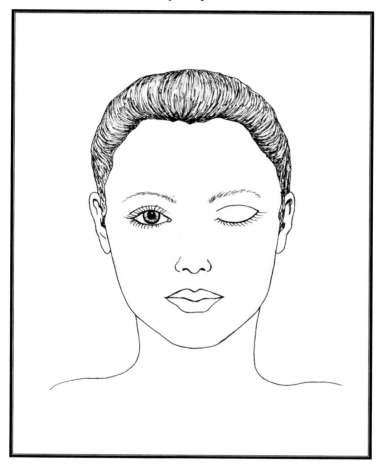

Your favourite products and colours:

Makeup	Brand	Colour
Foundation		
Lipstick		
Lip Liner		
Eye Shadow		
Eyeliner		

STRONG YIN: Cool, pure and strong blue tones

Strong's – skin often looks sallow and appears yellow. Rosy cheeks are seldom and they are usually quite pale. Cosmetics can improve their appearance dramatically! A common eye pattern resembles spokes of a wheel radiating from a hub (iris).

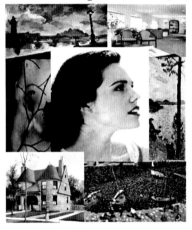

Hair Colour can be
Platinum blonde, (rare)
Salt and pepper, (black and white)
Medium to dark ash brown
Dark brown, (red highlights)
Black or brown/black, or blue/black
White or silver grey, (often premature)

Eye Colours can be
Blue or green with flecks
Grey/blue or Grey/green
dark blue or blue/violet
Turquoise or green/blue
Hazel, (brown near pupil + blue or green)
Dark rosy brown; black/brown

Skin Colouration can be
White or alabaster
White with delicate pink ton
Beige, (pale and often swallow)
Light, to deep rose beige
Olive, (beige/grey)

The swatch that appears best is silver, as it seems to add a youthful glow to the skin and eyes of the colours. Conversely, a yellow, sickly appearance happens when the gold cloth is next to the skin.

Strong Yin - coloured individuals are also the only ones that can wear true blue/black. I know most people love to wear black thinking that it is a sliming colour. The reality is that people with this colouring only, appear youthful and alive while others of different colouring will look washed out. The reason for this is that *Strong Yin Coloured* people have a high contrast between their hair, eyes and skin. No other colouring has more contrast!

Your Power Colour Charts

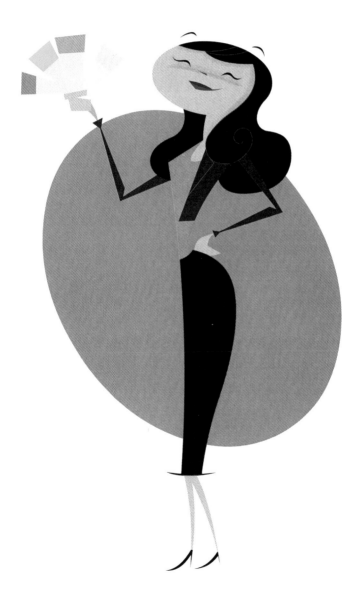

Colour Work sheet #1

Match your 36"x36" colour swatches (described on p. 50) to the following
Colour Harmonics Power Neutrals to determine where you sit on
the Yin / Yang colour scale.
YIN: Black 6 = Strong; #437 = Subtle // *YANG:* #478 = Deep; #466 = Bright

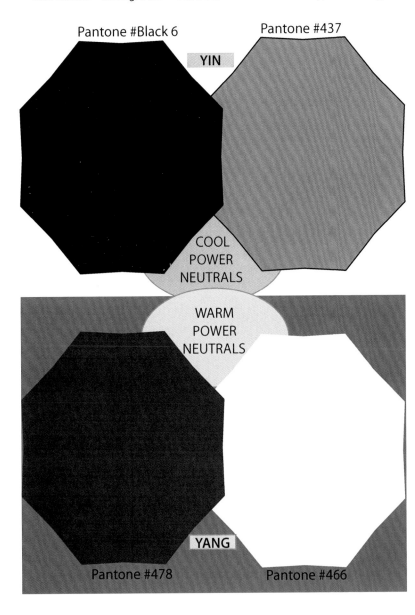

Pantone #Black 6

Pantone #437

YIN

COOL
POWER
NEUTRALS

WARM
POWER
NEUTRALS

YANG

Pantone #478

Pantone #466

Colour Work sheet #2

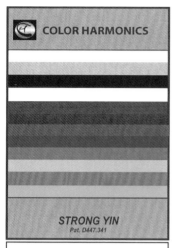

STRONG YIN
Pat. D447.341

*Skin often looks swallow, appears yellow & seldom has rosy cheeks
*A common eye pattern resembles spokes of a wheel radiating from a hub (iris).

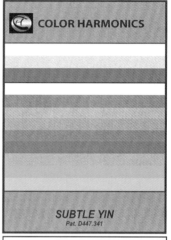

SUBTLE YIN
Pat. D447.341

*Skin is often thin or translucent.
* The blue undertone is easier to see and can have visible pink in skin.
* Eyes often have a cloudy, cracked-glass look.

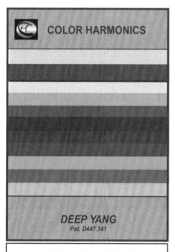

DEEP YANG
Pat. D447.341

*Pale beige or sallow, without rosy cheeks
*Peach-colored skin, can be florid or ruddy.
*No true blue eyes

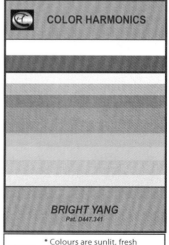

BRIGHT YANG
Pat. D447.341

* Colours are sunlit, fresh
* Clarity is the key
* Colours should be either delicate or vivid, never muted or dark.

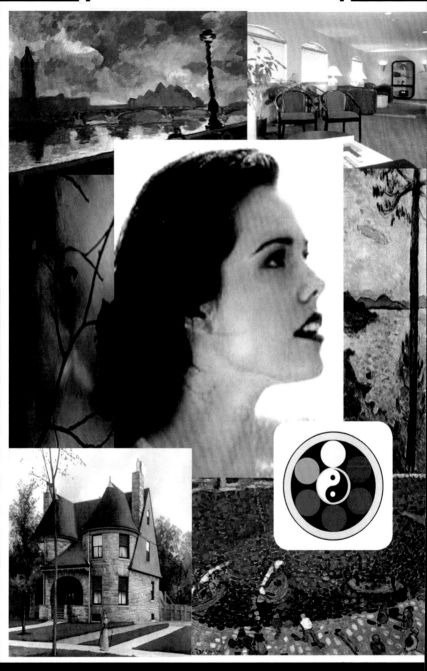

STRONG YIN

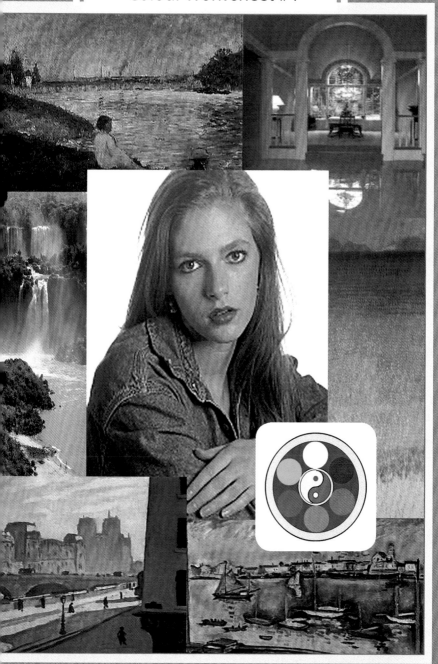

SUBTLE YIN

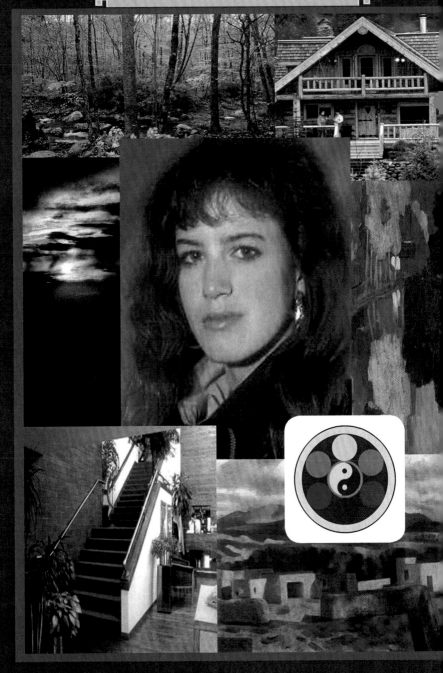

DEEP YANG

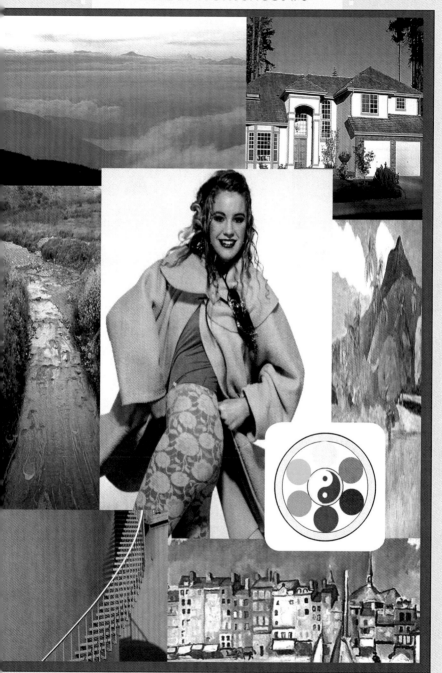

BRIGHT YANG

THE FOUR MAKEUP STYLES:

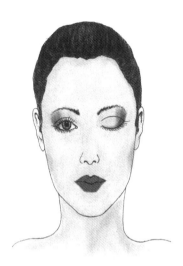

POLISHED STYLE

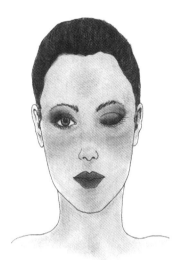

NATURAL STYLE

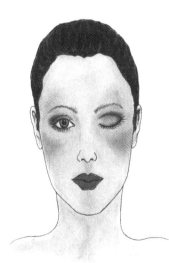

CLASSIC STYLE

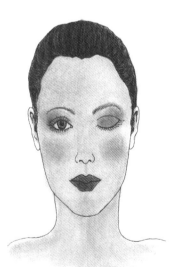

ARTISTIC STYLE

makeup colors shown are from the Strong Yin pallet

SUBTLE YIN: Cool, blended and dusted blue tones

Subtle's - have a blended appearance between their features - eyes, hair and skin. Their skin is often thin or translucent. They blush easily. Their eyes often have a cloudy, cracked glass look. The bluish undertone is easier to see on a *Subtle Yin* - than on a *Strong Yin,* and they can have visible pink in skin. These individuals use all five hues of colour but with a dusty blue undertone. They look the best in soft, pastel colours.

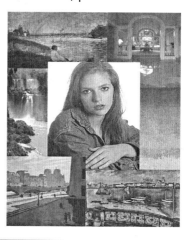

Hair Colour can be
light to dark ash blonde
brown with ash highlights
golden ash blonde (from the sun)
blue-gray or silver gray
pearly white or salt and pepper

Eye Colours can be
gray/blue or pale gray
blue or green - cloudy looking
blue or green - clear with white flecks
gray/green; bright clear blue
hazel, (brown with blue, or green)
aqua - clear, changes from green to blue

Skin Colouration can be
pale beige with pink cheeks
pale beige, (can be sallow)
rose beige, fair to deep

The swatch of silver appears considerably better on a *Subtle Yin - Coloured* individual than the gold. The only other swatch of the four noted that looks best on them is the Mauve taupe-coloured swatch. The reason: blue-based, blended colours enhance the subtle blue undertone in their skin and mavue-taupe is a colour clustered with blue undertones.

DEEP YANG: Warm, Deep and Saturated

Deep's – are often pale beige or sallow. Without rosy cheeks, they need blush. There are no true blue eyes in Deep Yang individuals. In the Deep Yang palette, warm golden undertones prevail and harmonize best.
Deep Yangs colours are deep, dusty, and saturated with gold. They have *Blended Colouring* with little contrast between hair, eye and skin colour.

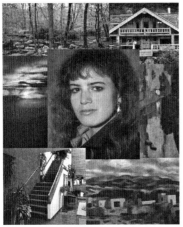

Hair Colour can be
strawberry blonde
honey or golden blonde
dirty blonde to Golden brown
deep chestnut brown
light to dark brown, with gold or red highlights
red to deep auburn
charcoal brown, or black
golden gray, or warm white

Skin Colouration can be
ivory, (also with freckles)
golden beige, (light to dark)
peach (light), to deep peach, (also with freckles)
coppery beige

Eye Colours can be
Olive green
Blue with teal or turquoise
Green - pale and clear
Hazel or amber
Golden brown
Dark brown

In the *Deep Yang* palette, warm golden undertones prevail and harmonize best. The swatch that reveals this best is the gold metallic swatch. Only a true *Deep Yang* looks good in root beer brown.

These people have a more blended *Colouring*; meaning that there is little contrast between hair, eye and skin colour. Therefore, they look best in rich dusty colours with, golden undertones.

BRIGHT YANG: Warm, Clear and Bright

Bright – coloured individuals have high contrast between the skin, hair and eyes. Therefore, colours of higher contrast with a yellow undertone, harmonize best on this person. *Bright Yang* colours are sunlit, fresh and radiant. Clarity is the key. Colours should be either vivid or delicate, not muted or dark.

Hair Colour can be
honey golden blonde
flaxen blonde, strawberry blonde
red auburn
golden brown, light to dark
golden grey, creamy white

Eye Colours can be
aqua or blue green
blue with white rays, (appear steel grey)
clear blue or green, (may have flecks)
hazel, (golden brown, green and gold)
light golden brown, or topaz

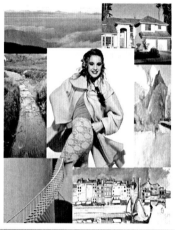

Skin Colouration can be
ivory, (also with freckles)
beige to golden beige
peach / pink (also with freckles)

The metallic gold swatch, when put around a *Bright Yang* - coloured person, highlights their eye and skin colour, which indicates a warm (yellow) undertone.

The next colour swatch, (out of the four chosen) that accents a *Bright Yang* - coloured person, is the wheat yellow.

With this individual, you will see a high contrast between the skin, hair and eyes. Therefore, colours of higher contrast and a yellow undertone, harmonize best on this person. Many of these individuals like to wear black but it isn't the best colour for them unless they wear khaki not blue-toned black.

Fill in your Personal Colouring information:

Your favourite colour is: _____
If you were to pack for a vacation for two weeks with only three colours to mix and match, what would they be?
1. _____   2._____   3._____

Your Skin Colour: _____
Your Eye Colour: _____
Your Natural Hair Colour: _____

Do you have:
Blended Colouring: _____ Or,
High Contrast Colouring: _____

Which metallic colour swatch makes your eyes come alive?
Gold ____ Silver ____

Which plain coloured cloth looks best?
Jet Black ___ Mauve Taupe___Wheat Yellow ___ Root Beer Brown ____

Which Colour Harmonic Group do you fit into?

Strong Yin: has *cool blue* undertone to skin. Use all five hues of colours with blue undertone. Primary colours along with clear, blue, and vivid colours look best. You have the *highest contrast* between hair, skin and eyes.

Subtle Yin: has *soft blue* undertone to skin. Use all five hues of colours with a dusted blue undertone. Use soft, pastel colours. You have *Blended Colouring* between hair, skin and eyes.

Deep Yang: has **warm** *golden* **undertone** to skin. Use all five hues of colours with golden yellow undertone. Use rich, mellow colours. *Blended Colouring* between hair, skin and eyes.

Bright Yang: has **warm** *yellow* **undertone** to skin. Use all five hues of colours with a clear yellow base. Use bright, clear colours. **High contrast** between hair, skin & eyes.

Your **Colour Harmonic Group** is:_____

THE PERFECT BODY IS DIVIDED INTO FOUR EQUAL PARTS

No Body is Perfect....

Your body is unique. By taking accurate measurements you will know what type of clothing will best enhance your particular structure or body shape.

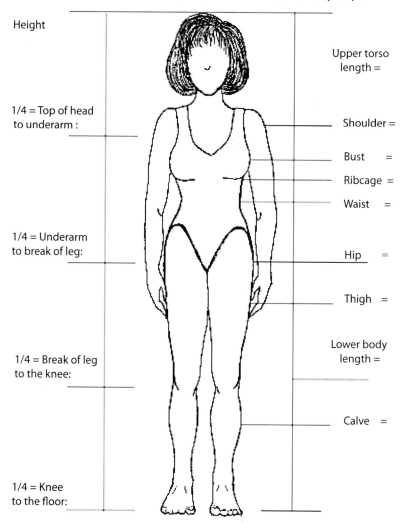

Height

Upper torso
length =

1/4 = Top of head
to underarm :

Shoulder =

Bust   =

Ribcage =

Waist   =

1/4 = Underarm
to break of leg:

Hip   =

Thigh   =

Lower body
length =

1/4 = Break of leg
to the knee:

Calve   =

1/4 = Knee
to the floor:

Fill in your measurements here for a visual record of your body shape.

How do you measure up?

Your Height:
Top of the head to Hip Bone (pivot joint):   _____
Hip Bone to the Floor: _____
            I have _____ Legs.

Waist Line Measurement:
Measure from the crease of the underarm to hipbone: _____
Natural waist indentation - from your underarm to your waist: _____
From waist to your hip bone (pelvic hinge bone):   _____
            I have a _____ Waist.

Hips and Waist:
Bust Measurement: _____
Waist Measurement: _____
Hip Measurement - (fullest part at pivot bone):   _____

            I have _____Hips. (Average, small, large)

On an average body, the hips will measure 2" more than the bust, and 9-10" more than the waist.

Bust Measurement:
Pull tape across fullest part of breasts and straight across your back: _____
The chest measurement just below the breast is: _____
Subtract this measurement from the first: _____

            I am Small // Average // Large busted. I need a size _____bra

If bust measurement is less than 1" larger than chest measurement = you are Small.
If measurement is 1-3" larger than chest measurement = your bust size is Average.
If measurement is larger than 3" of chest size = you are Large.
This is a guide to cup size: *Small* - "A" cup; *Average* - "B or C" cup; *Large* - "D" cup or larger

Shoulder Measurement:
The circumference of the shoulder relative to the hips is:
Circumference of shoulders: _____
Circumference of hips: _____

            I have _____SHOULDERS.

Consider equal width of shoulders to width of hips = *Average.*
Wider shoulder measurement than hips = *Broad Shoulders.*
Shoulders that are less than hip measure = *Narrow Shoulders.*

The "CLOTHES CLOCK" tells your LIFESTYLE

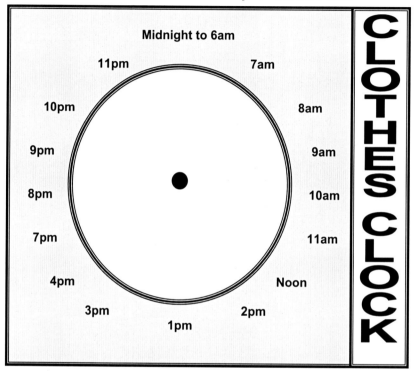

Use as many *minute & hour* arrows, filled in-between with the following GRID. This *tells* you where you spend the MOST TIME in a day and *tells* you what TYPE & STYLE of CLOTHES you should spend the MOST MONEY on when purchasing a new wardrobe.

CASUAL WEAR

DRESSY CASUAL

WORK WEAR

FORMAL WEAR

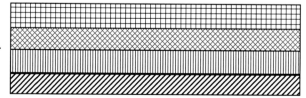

FOOLPROOF WARDROBE PLANNING

At this point, you know your **Dominant Inner-trait, Colour Ruler, and what your Body and Face Shape** is. You also know your **Clothes Clock needs**. It's time to build your working wardrobe.

A basic wardrobe plan uses '*SEPARATES*' that '*COORDINATE*'.
Choose 2 or 3 Basic Colours from your Colour Ruler.
List three of your Colour Harmonic Power Colours:

1. _____
2. _____
3. _____

2 + 2 + 5 = > 48 COORDINATING OUTFITS

2   Solid colour suits   (= two matching skirts & jackets)
+
2   Pants or skirts   (= Solid ¶ or, patterned #)
+
5   Tops   (= blouse + top + sweater + cardigan + jacket)

≥   48 Coordinated Outfits

The chart below displays the colour number and pattern symbol of clothing items in your closet right now. On the next page, place the colours numbers to create a successful working wardrobe.

Two Suits	Two Pants	Two Skirts
A	A	A
B	B	B

Combine with any of the following: *use the key below to identify your needs*

Blouse	Top	Sweater	Cardigan	Jacket

KEY: ☺ - Have >   * - Need >   ?- Want >

CLOSET INVENTORY SHEET

_____ **Working Wardrobe:**

(*) Already own the item   **(!)** need the item now
(?) want the item soon

COLOURS	JACKETS	SKIRT/DRESS	PANTS	BLOUSES
A B C D				
NAVY				
GREY				
YELLOW				
ORANGE				
RED				
GREEN				
BLUE				

*All clothes selected in the chart above should harmonize
with the following category that was selected.

A = Black / White   Strong Yin
B = Taupe / Off White   Subtle Yin
C = Camel / Ivory   Bright Yang
D = Brown / Beige   Deep Yang

Notes:

Your Personal Working Wardrobe - Key Sheet

< 50 COLOUR COORDINATING OUTFITS

CLOTHING ITEM	COLOUR	COMBINES WITH
Jacket	Basic Colour #1	All skirts and pants
Jacket	Basic Colour #2	All skirts and pants
Skirt	Basic Colour #1	All tops and jackets
Skirt	Basic Colour #2	All tops and jackets
Skirt	Basic Colour #1	Most jackets & blouses
Skirt	Coordinate #1, #2	All jackets and blouses
Blouse (solid colour)	Basic or #3 accent	All skirts, pants, jackets
Blouse (solid colour)	Basic Colour #1	All skirts, pants, jackets
Blouse (solid colour)	Basic Colour #2	Most skirts, pants, jackets
Top (solid colour)	Accent colour #3	All skirts, pants, jackets
Soft-Structured Jacket	Accent colour #3	All skirts, pants, jackets

Accessories:

SHOES	PURSES	BELTS
Pumps #1 / # 2	Clutch #1 / # 2	Leather dressy
Sandals #1 / #2 / #3	Shoulder #1 / #2 / #3	Fabric with loop
Flats #1 / #2 / #3	Oversize #1	Leather casual
Boots #1	Evening #1 or #3	Chain

Other: Fragrance / Hair adornments / Jewellery / Makeup

Complete the above tables and you have a *basic* working wardrobe.

Your Personal Style Journal

Name: _____

Mailing Address: _____

City: _____Prov/State: _____

Country: _____ Postal/Zip : _____-_____

Email: _____

Personal Colouring: _____

Main Colour Preference: _____

Secondary: _____

Your Body Shape: _____

Body Shape Challenge: _____

Face Shape: _____

Challenge: _____

Clothing Personality:_____

Secondary: _____

Clothes Clock: Suit Types: Dressy:

Casual: Dressy /Casual:

Clothing Challenges: _____

Personality Type: _____

Secondary: _____

Conclusion

At the beginning, I stated that this concept also transformed into your Interior Style.It does.If you watch any decorating shows on TV today you are sure to have heard terms like French Country, Traditional Tudor; Contemporary; Country Chic; Neo Classic; Modern or Transitional.It is enough to make your head swim!

For the average person whose life revolves around more than their house décor, simple and more effective terms that I like to use describe *Shapes* that reflect what you like rather than *Style* terms to tell you who you are. Your personality does that.

I use the same four shape terms to discover and display your style.They are Straight; Substantial; Symmetrical and Spherical and Synchronistic. OK, how do those words make Interior Design any easier? Well, for one thing you start with a clean palette for imaging a room that you would love to live in.If I told you that you leaned towards a Country Style.What did you just see in your head? Appliance cozies, bunches of dried flowers and gingham curtains? Maybe I meant South American Country – new image? See the problem?

OK, try this instead.Picture the word *Straight*. What comes to mind – minimal, simple, clean lines without a lot of adornment or fuss? Form before function is the best way to describe this.

Now picture the word *Substantial*.What picture did you create in your head? Possibly did the shapes have bulkier lines with blunt rather than sharp edges and maybe larger in scale? Here function and comfort leads form.

Let's try another one seeing how we are getting the hang of this.*Symmetrical* – easy right? Not too large, nor too small; not too sharp or blunt. A shape that is somewhat stylized with adornments. Balanced is the key word here.

How about *Spherical?* Do you see rounded, free flowing shapes that transcend structure and push the limits in both materials used and sometimes even taste! Getting the idea?

Finally the term *Eclectic* – a much misused term whose real definition is the best of all periods and styles harmonized together as a unit through correct use of scale, colour and mood. I refer to this as *Synchronistic Style* where "Feng-tional" harmony in all living spaces is strived for regardless of style terms used today. Your home after all is your rejuvenation place. Make it you!

Look for *Discovering your Interior Style - 8 Steps to Design Diva* to learn how to create your own personal and unique decorating style.

If you are thinking of or have started your own business venture, then Discovering your Industry Style - 8 steps to Business Branding would help you move your image to your interior and industry style to make sure your are attracting the right target market. This book completes the series of the Triple ID Style Classification System.

Time to look in the mirror.

Congratulations G.U.R.U. You have Discovered Your Inner Style.

- GEE YOU ARE YOU - live, authentic and true! Now go and Express it!

Suggested Reading Materials

Books on the importance of colour:

Colour: Universal Language & Dictionary Of Names, US Dept. Of Commerce (National Bureau Of Standards). NBC Special Publication 440.

Colour Psychology & Colour Therapy: Faber Birren University Books, New Hyde Park, NY, 1961.

Colour Therapy: The Ancient Art Of, Linda Clark, The Devin-Adair Company Old Greenwich, Connecticut.

Colour Me Beautiful: Carol Jackson, Acropolis, Washington, D.C., 1980.

Colour Your World: Frank Don, Van Nostrand Reinhold Co. NY, 1982.

Light, Colour & Environment: Revised Edition, Faber Birren, Van Nostrand Reinhold Co., NY, 1982.

Living Colour: Sarah Rossbach And Lin Yun, Kodansha America, Inc. 1994.

Principles Of Colour: Faber Birren, Van Nostrand Reinhold Co., New York, NY, 1969.

Principles Of Colour Technology: 2nd Edition, Fred W. Billlmeyer Jr. And Max Saltzman, John Wiley & Son, New York, NY, 1981.

The Luscher Colour Test: Scot Ian, Pocket Books New York, NY, 1971.

The Psychology Of Colour & Design: Deborah T. Sharpe, Nelson-Hall Co. Chicago, Ill. 1974.

Books on image & wardrobe planning:

Clothes Sense: Barbara Weiland And Leslie Wood, Palmer And Pletsch, Portland, Oregon, 1984.

Look, Working & Living Terrific 24 Hours A Day: Emily Cho And Hermine Lueders, Putnam's & Sons, New York, NY, 1982.

Metamorphosis: David Kibbe, Macmillan Publishing Company New York, NY, 1987.

The Woman's Dress For Success: John T. Malloy, Follett 1977. Also In Paperback By Warner Books 1978.

The Lutterloh International System: Modeverlag Lutterloh Mcmlxxiv - P.o. Box 3149, D-8990 Lindau, W. Germany.

Working Wardrobe: Janet Wallach, Acropolis Books, In Washington, D.C., 1981.

Face Reading Secrets: Rose Rosetree, Ottenheimer Publishers, Baltimore, Maryland, 1994.

Personality Plus: By Florence Litteraur.

The Celestine Prophecy: James Redfield, Warner Books, Inc. New York, NY, 1993.

Understanding Human Behavior: (Text) BPC Publishing Ltd, Distributed By Columbia House New York, NY, 1974.

Books On Psychology:

Do What You Are: Paul D. Tieger And Barbara Barron-Tieger, Little, Brown & Co., 1992.

Modern Man In Search Of A Soul By C.G. Jung Translated By Ws Dell And Carl F. Baynes, Harcourt Brace Jovananich, Orlando, Florida.

Carl Rogers On Personal Power By Carl R. Rogers Phd., Delacorte Press, New York, NY, 1977.

Understanding Psychological Research: Marion Lewis.

Public Appearance And Private Realities: Mark Snyder, Wh Freeman And Co. New York, NY, 1986.

Books On Interior Design Styles:

Better Homes & Gardens New Decorating Book: Meredith Corporation, Des Moines, Iowa, 1990.

The House & Garden Book Of Romantic Rooms: Robert Harling And Leonie Highton And John Bridges, William Collins & Sons Co. Ltd., 1985.

Laura Ashley - Complete Guide To Home Decorating: Harmony Books, New York, NY.

The Feng Shui House Book: Change Your Home Transform Your Life Gina Lazenby, Raincoast Books, Vancouver, BC, Canada, 1998.

Favourite Websites:
www.colormatters.com - Interesting colour facts and theories

www.pantone.com - Where colour comes from and is used personally and in industry

www.bodybuilding.com/fun/becker3.htm - Discuss Ectomorph, Mesomorph and Endomorph body type theories.

www.yumieto.com - Makes clothing to fit different body shapes

www.aboutfaceimage.com - Deborah Reynolds, an amazing image consultant.

www.phreshspa.com - Kimberly Pettifer, pHresh Spa & Wellness Club in Vancouver, BC

www.salonweb.com - Discusses face shapes and give hairstyle tips.

www.visual-makeover.com - Gives tips on Hair styles

www.hair-styles.org - Hair style photos for face shapes

www.simplyproductive.com - Sherry Borsheim, a Professional Organizer for home and office

www.kickstartcommunications.com - Cathrine Levan – a 'butt kicking' publishing agent that gets you to your goal

www.diamondstarcoaching.com -Laurel Hillton an amazing and dynamic personal and business coach

Testimonials

In love, opposites attract, but in designing and furnishing a home this romantic notion is just a dream. Fortunately, Jan Addams' approach to design made this sometimes painful and frustrating process easy and insightful! My husband and I are now happily snuggled, in our nice and cosy little home, reflection both our tastes, and personalities.

-Judith Pilsner Bed. BFA, Fort McMurray, AB.

For an interior design illiterate, and one whose main passions lie elsewhere, this book has been perfect for me. In a clear, concise, straightforward manner, this very interesting book has pulled together all the facets of one's colouring, personality, and psyche (also that of the whole family unit), to ensure the total flowing. I have had the pleasure of experiencing firsthand, the creativeness of Ms. Addams, watching with trepidation and then glee, as shoe tore my home apart, and then put it back together so effortlessly and elegantly. Thank you Ms. Addams. This book has taken so much fear away.

-B. Johnson, Lethbridge, AB

Inside Out Image to Interior by Janice E. Addams. This course is an inside look into you as an individual: putting a finger on why we make the colour and style choices that we do. It shows the individual how to put their own personality into their homes and works spaces. In short, understanding our personal style can bring a balance to our life.

-Coleen Sexsmith-Gagnon, Interior Designer, Calgary, Alberta

Image to Interior Products

NOTE: ALL PRICES IN CANADIAN DOLLARS

qty:	item:	price:
_____	Personal Colour tags ....$ 5.95	
_____	Your Style Cards ....$ 24.95	
_____	Colour Harmonics Tool..$ 15.95	
_____	Discovering Your Inner Style.....................................$ 24.95	

For more information or to place an order today
CALL
or Email
info@imagetointerior.com

TOTAL ORDER (CAN $): _____

Quantity discounts available.
Shipping/Handling not included.

Name: _____

Address: _____

City: _____ Prov/State: _____

Country: _____ Postal/Zip Code: _____

Phone: (_____) _____ Email: _____

Charge my _____**VISA** _____**Mastercard**

Card Number: _____

Exp Date: _____ Name on Card: _____

Signature: _____

Mail orders please send to:
Box 309 3495 Cambie Street
Vancouver BC V5Z 4E3

Please allow
4–6 weeks
for delivery.

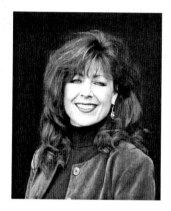

Janice E Addams MIRM is both an Interior Designer and an Interior Merchandiser (MIRM). MIRM is the top-level achievement for professionals in the new home industry. Over the last decade, she has used her varied education to interior design and merchandise 100's of model homes Dozens of those same homes have been featured in local papers and builder magazines. Many have gone on to win the coveted SAM Awards (Sales & Marketing Awards of Excellence).

Jan uses her talent, vision, and education to create interior design plans that reflect the occupant's image style not her style. Jan's mandate is to "de-stress, not distress" her clients. The Triple ID Style Classification System© was developed to help simplify the interior design selection process. It uses the client's own personal colouring, body type and personality to create an interior design style that is as individual and unique as each client serviced. Jan uses computer assisted 3D design programs to give her clients a visual idea of what the proposed design project will look like before any construction starts. Information is relayed via email, fax or in person. Everything possible is done to help create a sense of trust and comfort in the planning, design, building or renovating process of a home, office or commercial space.

Image to Interior Inc. is an innovative and progressive image to interior design & merchandising firm whose objective is to facilitate the successful execution of projects from "concept to completion."

The firm is located in the beautiful province of British Columbia, Canada and utilizes the superb talent of many local professionals and trades' people; general contractors, tile setters, cabinet makers, mill workers, upholsterers, seamstresses, blind and window covering creators and installers; painters, artists, artisans as well as photographers and videographers to bring the finished design job to life.